STOP A.D.D. NATURALLY

Breakthrough Information About
Amino Acid and Vitamin Therapy
That Can Change Your Child's Life!

By Billie Jay Sahley, Ph.D., C.N.C.

Foreword by Doris Rapp, M.D.

Pain & Stress Publications®
San Antonio, Texas
July 2003

Note to Readers

This material is not intended to replace the services of a physician, nor is it meant to encourage diagnosis and treatment of illness, disease, or other medical problems by the layperson. This book should not be regarded as a substitute for professional medical treatment, and while every care is taken to ensure the accuracy of the content, the author and the publishers cannot accept legal responsibility for any problem arising out of experimentation with the methods described. Any application of the recommendations set forth in the following pages is at the reader's discretion and sole risk. If you are under a physician's care for any condition, he or she can advise you whether the program described in this book is suitable for you or your child. If your child is taking Ritalin or other medication, DO NOT STOP the medication without a physician's assistance.

No part of this publication may be reproduced, stored in a retrieval system, or transmitted in any form or by any means electronic, mechanical, photocopied, recorded, or otherwise without the prior written permission of the author.

This publication has been compiled through research resources at the Pain & Stress Center, San Antonio, Texas.

The names of the patients described in this book have been changed to protect their privacy.

Fifth Edition, Pain & Stress Publications®
July 2003

Additional copies may be ordered from:
Pain & Stress Center Products
5282 Medical Drive, Suite 160, San Antonio, Texas 78229-5379
1-800-669-2256

Library of Congress Catalog Control Number 2003108477
ISBN 1-889391-24-7

Acknowledgments

My sincere appreciation and thanks to:

The staff of the Pain & Stress Center for their dedication to helping children. A special thanks to Linda Volpenhein, C.N.C., for all her extra effort and contributions to helping children with special needs.

Antonio L. Ruiz, M.D., Medical Director of the Pain & Stress Center, for his support.

Dr. Katherine M. Birkner for her scientific collaboration that helped make this book possible.

Doris Rapp, M.D., one of God's gifted healers, and an inspiration to those who reach out to the hyperactive children of the world.

Sherry Rogers, M.D., for opening the doors to life's most important mineral, magnesium chloride.

To the many parents of hyperactive children who believed in me and encouraged my research in the role of amino acids and nutrients in brain functioning and behavior.

The new generation of physicians, therapists, and educators who seek natural alternatives through nutritional medicine.

To the *Lord for always lighting my path.*

Contents

Tryptophan	Magnesium	Vitamin C
5-HTP	Calcium	Vitamin E
GABA	Zinc	Liquid Serotonin
L-Glutamine	Chromium	Huperzine
Taurine	B Vitamins	Phosphatidylserine
Tyrosine	Niacinamide	Vinpocetine
Glycine	Pyridoxine (B6)	

Charts/Special Information

Note to the Reader:

In some cases, the author has referred to a child as "him." Ordinarily she would take every measure to use nongender language. But, in view of the fact that most A.D.D./A.D.H.D. children are young boys, she is comfortable using male gender identification.

Foreword

In the 1930s Dr. Rowe reported hyperactivity in children could be due to foods. In the 1940s revealed chemicals as a definite cause of learning and activity problems. Dr. Spear in the 1950s coined the term, Allergic-Tension-Fatigue Syndrome—attributing it to the common allergens such as dust, molds, pollen, and foods. Children exhibiting these same symptoms during the last thirty years were diagnosed with A.D.D. or A.D.H.D. Today, A.D.D. or A.D.H.D. is the "in" diagnosis.

Twenty years ago, any experienced teacher would have told you, a child rarely needed a drug for over activity. Today physicians report the immune system, endocrine, reproductive, and nervous systems are weaker than ever. Why?

- Why has this happened?
- What have we done wrong?
- How can we correct it?

Genetically, I believe we are not as strong as we once were. Today, there is an epidemic of new allergies—allergies, illnesses, and chemical sensitivities. Rare medical problems such as cancer are now rampant. Learning disabilities, depression, mood and behavior problems are increasing at an unbelievable rate.

What have we done wrong? One cause is the increased use of harmful chemicals and pesticides in our air, food, and water. I personally believe this is one factor related to our present epidemic of hyperactivity and A.D.D. Are the elevated pesticide levels in milk (cow and breast) one reason why infants manifest obvious hyperactivity? We must help our children by reducing chemicals in our foods, air, water, clothing, and houses so that we do not harm their brains and bodies.

We need more rational approaches to help the children who are out of control or hyperactive. Even if a parent's medical insurance covers the cost of a Class II narcotic drug such as Ritalin, it is my belief that all parents, at least initially, consider more natural approaches to hyperactivity. Why are we using drugs that are harmful when proper nutrients—amino acids and vitamins, natural diet, and homeopathies support the brain and body and are not harmful. Most parents do not realize the potential side effects that occur with activity-modifying drugs. We must find out why children display hyperactive behavior—and avoid mind-altering drugs.

What else can you do? Educate and inform yourself. Learn all you can about hyperactivity and A.D.D. This small, but most comprehensive book is a true gem—containing an immense number of valuable and sensible insights, solutions, and explanations. Dr. Sahley clearly explains exactly what needs to improve and restore the brain chemistry of our children. Orthomolecular therapy treats each child or adult's individual needs. Dr. Sahley has diligently formulated precise formulas for children with specific medical, learning, and activity problems. These formulas provide practical, sensible help. We should all be grateful that Dr. Sahley has the dedication, insight, and knowledge to develop formulas to help A.D.D. or A.D.H.D. children.

So curl up in your favorite chair—and don't just read this book, but study it so you can help your child and yourself. You can't change the entire world, but you can help your child think more clearly, behave more appropriately, and enjoy life more fully! Once you see how much this book helps, share it with others—so we can help more children without using mind-altering drugs. That's what life is really all about. Give and share as much as you can to help as many as possible.

> Bless you,
> Doris Rapp, M.D.

What is Hyperactivity?

The following definition excerpts from the book, *Toxic Psychiatry,* by Peter B. Breggin, M.D., noted psychiatrist in private practice and a past consultant with the *National Institute of Mental Health.*

"Hyperactivity is the most frequent justification for drugging children. The difficult-to-control male child is certainly not a new phenomenon, but attempts to give him a medical diagnosis are the product of modern psychology and psychiatry. At first psychiatrists called hyperactivity a brain disease. When no brain disease could be found, they changed it to 'minimal brain disease' (MBD). When no minimal brain disease could be found, the profession transformed the concept into minimal brain dysfunction. When no minimal brain dysfunction could be demonstrated, the label became attention deficit disorder. Now it's just assumed no real disease, regardless of the failure to prove it so."

Noted psychiatrist, Abram Hoffer, M.D., Ph.D., states, "You can take this same difficult child to ten psychiatrists and come back with ten different diagnoses. But no matter what the diagnosis is, they all put him on Ritalin. Psychiatry is the one branch where the diagnosis means nothing because it doesn't determine treatment. Nutritional deficiencies must be addressed. If a doctor is not a good nutritionist, he cannot be a good physician." Dr. Hoffer is recognized for his landmark discoveries in the fields of psychiatry and medicine. He has written several books, including *Orthomolecular Medicine for Physicians.* Dr. Hoffer serves as editor-in-chief of the *Journal of Orthomolecular Medicine.*

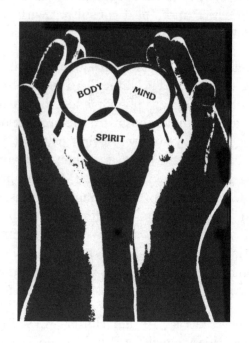

Introduction

Orthomolecular therapy means supplying the cells with the right mixture of nutrients. Many diseases result from the wrong balance of essential nutrients in the body. Adjusting the diet, eliminating junk foods, and ingesting the proper doses of essential vitamins, minerals, and amino acids can correct the chemical imbalances.

The orthomolecular approach helps patients become more aware of our dangerously polluted environment and nutrient-stripped refined foods. The orthomolecular approach is both corrective and preventive. Meganutrient therapy has become a part of orthomolecular medicine. While becoming widely recognized that orthomolecular therapy helps people by correcting the brain's chemical imbalances, little is known that certain meganutrient combinations can be as immediately effective as potent painkillers or tranquilizers. Meganutrients treat the person's whole biochemical imbalances. They can provide immediate and long-term benefit. The type of treatment offered by orthomolecular doctors and therapists varies, but the mainstream of work focuses upon meganutrient therapy, diagnostic tests, and treatment with adequate nutrients—a distinguishing characteristic of orthomolecular medicine.

Orthomolecular therapy considers every individual to be biochemically unique. Every person requires a very different combination of nutrients and amino acids. Application of this therapy meets each individual's need, and the mind and body reach a state of homeostasis. Homeostasis is a condition where everything in the body is in balance and capable of resisting environmental changes, while regulating internal metabolic functions.

Nutrition affects every cell in the body. When nutrition

is inadequate, the kidneys stop filtering, the stomach stops digesting, the adrenals stop secreting, and soon the other organs follow suit.

Good nutrition is the preservation of health and prevention of disease—especially with respect to the question of optimum intake of essential vitamins, minerals, and amino acids. New breakthroughs in nutritional science give parents hope for a world beyond Ritalin. The late Dr. Roger Williams from the University of Texas Clayton Foundation, through his research, opened new doors into understanding the brain's chemistry and the use of amino acids. Dr. Williams' research demonstrated that, for maximum function, the brain must be constantly nourished. The brain never sleeps—it is a 24-hour power source. Yet, the brain is the most undernourished organ in the body. Nourishment, not Ritalin, provides the answer for the millions of children in the U.S. who are given this powerful amphetamine—a form of speed—everyday. Ritalin is habit forming and causes over sixteen adverse side effects that are listed in the *P.D.R. (Physician's Desk Reference).*

Ritalin, or any other amphetamine, tranquilizer, or antidepressant, cannot give the brain or body nourishment. C.H.A.D.D. (Children with Attention Deficit Disorder), a parents' organization that promotes the use of Ritalin to drug their children and themselves, is currently conducting public relations and lobbying the FDA to remove Ritalin as a Schedule II drug. Schedule II drugs are those the Drug-Enforcement-Agency (DEA) lists as having the highest potential for abuse. Should this happen, the children in this country will not have a chance to live just as kids, to laugh, or even cry. We were not born with Ritalin in our brains, *so how can we be Ritalin deficient?*

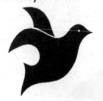

A.D.D. and Hyperactivity

Approximately 6 million children in this country suffer some type of learning disability, hyperactivity, A.D.D. (Attention Deficit Disorder), or hyperkinesis. More than two million children currently take Ritalin for A.D.D. and A.D.H.D. A.D.D. and A.D.H.D. may be caused by psychological problems, including trauma and abuse. Other causes could be physiological disorders such as nutritional deficiencies, chemical imbalances, blood sugar disturbances, allergic responses to food and chemicals, or a poor diet. A failure in the brain's inhibitory system—the ability of the brain to inhibit and control itself—may also causes A.D.D/A.D.H.D.

Ritalin is an amphetamine available by physician's prescription, and is prescribed daily for thousands of children who not only do not need Ritalin, but who will suffer from its effects mentally and physically. Prescription rates for Ritalin doubled between 1992 and 1996. The United States Drug Enforcement Administration lists five grades of controlled substances based on abuse potential. Heroin and LSD fall under Schedule I. Schedule II drugs include morphine, opium, and Ritalin. Yet this potent drug is being used as a quick fix to quiet children, whether the drug is needed or not.

Children who demonstrate symptoms of hyperkinesis, hyperactivity, or Attention Deficit Disorder could have an imbalance in their brain's biochemistry. A biochemical imbalance results from a deficiency of neurotransmitters, the chemical language of the brain. This deficiency affects the brain's inhibitory system. If a biochemical imbalance goes untreated, a child may display maladaptive behavior, followed by possible long-term physical and emotional problems.

A child's state of health reflects his or her state of

nutrition. When minerals, vitamins, amino acids, enzymes, or even hormones are deficient in a child's system, the result can be a disturbed biochemical homeostasis causing impaired functions in the brain. This, in turn, can cause an inability to focus, concentrate, and stay on task.

At the Pain and Stress Center in San Antonio, we have successfully treated numerous children with orthomolecular therapy. For the majority of cases, orthomolecular therapy corrects the brain's biochemical imbalance, without toxic drugs that can produce adverse side effects. Orthomolecular therapy corrects the child's biochemical imbalances that affect both short-term and long-term behaviors.

Each child receives a complete evaluation which includes food-sensitivity screening and an amino acid profile from blood work. The blood tests provide an effective means of revealing the offending foods and specific amino-acid deficiencies. In many cases foods eaten on a regular basis can cause numerous problems that can contribute to hyperactivity and A.D.D. behavior. These are known as hidden food sensitivities. The blood test uncovers hidden sensitivities and confirms which foods cause immediate or delayed reactions. The orthomolecular approach provides dietary reforms, amino acids, vitamins, and special nutrients to enhance the optimum molecular environment for each child's mind and body.

A.D.D./A.D.H.D. presents a major problem facing parents today. Most people think of hyperactivity as some type of behavioral problem—a child who is impatient, impulsive, and constantly moving; but not all hyperactive children are aggressive. Some are very passive, withdrawn, and find it hard to communicate their feelings.

Let's examine the list of passive and aggressive behaviors and see exactly where your child might fit in. Some children have multiple symptoms—they may display both passive and aggressive behaviors.

If your child demonstrates aggressive/passive behaviors,

Behavior Symptoms Displayed by Children with Hyperactivity or Attention Deficit Disorder

Aggressive

Angry outbursts *sometimes*
Quarrelsomeness *sometimes*
Aggressiveness *sometimes*
Restlessness *sometimes*
Stealing
Resentment of punishment *sure*
Unaware of danger(s)
Inability to concentrate *yes*
Self-mutilation
Compulsive aggression
Not good in sports *sometimes*
Temper tantrums *sometimes*
Unable to complete projects *sometimes*
Junk-food eater *sure*
High sugar and caffeine *NO*
  intake *(probably)*
Poor muscle coordination
Lying
Irregular sleep habits
Poor handwriting, drawing,
  and reading skills
Showoff attitude
Bully
Inability to make and keep
  friends

Passive

Depressed moods
Anxious *sometimes*
Fearful *sometimes*
Stays close to mother
Mood swings
Sleep problems
Withdrawn
Accident prone
Emotional instability *sometimes*
Distractibility *yes*
Crying spells *sometimes*
Poor math calculations *sometimes*
Daydreams *sure*
Eating problems
Poor muscle coordination
Lying
Headaches *sometimes*
Skin problems such as
  rash or hives *sometimes*
Reasoning difficulty *sometimes*
Poor reading skills
Hyperventilates
Poorly developed
  musculo-skeletal system
Insecurity *sometimes*
Shyness *sometimes*

keep a daily log for one month. This log should include stressful situations, increased anxiety, food cravings, and behavioral patterns. At the end of the month the log will help you understand your child's behavior and will provide valuable information should additional therapy be required.

Dr. Alan Gaby in an article in the *Townsend Letter for Doctors*, April 1994, states, "It is time to take a closer look at a possible relationship between attention deficit disorder, hyperactivity, and subclinical hypothyroidism." Dr. Gaby reports he has seen several hyperactive and A.D.D. children improve after taking a thyroid hormone. Ray Peat, Ph.D., confirms the same success as Dr. Gaby. Dr. Peat states, "For many years a few physicians have known about the quieting effects of thyroid, and have prescribed it for hyperactive children." According to Dr. Peat, thyroid hormones are essential for providing the energy to keep the brain at a high energy level all the time. This high energy level allows the frontal lobes of the brain to function at the needed performance level. If the child's system does not maintain this energy, attention span diminishes and the dominant behavior demonstrated includes stress, anxiety, and tension. If you suspect a thyroid problem, consult your physician for more information and blood tests. Use your daily log to describe the behavior patterns.

A.D.D./A.D.H.D. is not a condition that can be measured in precise scientific terms. Nor is it a situation with a quick fix, especially with a powerful and addictive drug such as Ritalin. A.D.D./A.D.H.D. is a complex and intricate condition in which children demonstrate maladaptive or disorganized behaviors that put them out of sync with the world around them. Because of their inadequacies, A.D.D./A.D.H.D. children prove extremely vulnerable to other people. Given this information, you must take into consideration his environment, food sensitivities, allergic reactions to foods, chemicals, poor diet, and brain chemistry, especially low levels of serotonin and inhibitory neurotransmitters.

The Ritalin Epidemic

Too many teachers pressure parents by telling them, "Your child is disrupting my class—maybe he should be put on Ritalin." Is this why U.S. manufacturers increased the production of Ritalin 62% in 1994? Teachers, especially, need to be educated about natural alternatives and nutrient deficiencies. They should educate and inform, not medicate and ignore.

Latest records from the manufacturers of Ritalin indicate approximately 4 million children now take it on a regular basis. Usage has more than doubled in the last seven years. According to Peter Breggin, M.D., in his book, *Talking Back to Ritalin: What Doctors Aren't Telling You about Stimulants for Children,* there were more than 2,700 "adverse drug experiences" filed to the FDA between 1985 and 1987 by pharmacologists and consumers. A report in the *Journal of the American Medical Association,* October 21, 1988, discusses a survey of school nurses in all county and private schools in the Baltimore area to determine the prevalence of medication treatment for hyperactivity/inattentiveness. The results reveal a consistent doubling every four to seven years of the rate of medicating treatment for hyperactive and inattentive students. The report shows 5.96% of all public elementary school students receiving such treatment. With all the research available documenting the long-term negative side effects of Ritalin, why won't educators educate themselves instead of requesting drugs! Not one of these educators would put their own children on Ritalin or any other psychotropic drug.

"In the late 1980's, the stimulant medication treatment of U.S. children has returned to become a noteworthy public issue" (*New York Times,* May 5, 1987, p. 3 and *The Reporter*

Weekly, September 2, 1987, p. 10). "If present trends continue, over 1 million U.S. children will be receiving stimulant medication by the early 1990's, or for inattentiveness associated with a learning impairment." The report continues to make an additional statement, "In view of this, additional public-health oriented assessment research should be funded." On May 5, 1987, the *New York Times* ran a story entitled, " Sales of Drug are Soaring for Treatment of Hyperactivity." The results of this soaring increase should include more specific guidelines for physicians! Prior to giving a prescription, physicians should inform and provide parents a list of the adverse side effects, as well as long-term effects of Ritalin. Physicians should inform parents that Ritalin is an addictive and strong stimulant with many adverse side effects. In some cases, Ritalin can produce the very symptoms it is suppose to control—increased hyperactivity, agitation, and impulsivity.

In the same journal Sally Shaywitz, M.D., and Bennett Shaywitz, M.D., of Yale University School of Medicine, wrote an editorial about Attention Deficit Hyperactivity Disorder (A.D.H.D.). A.D.H.D. represents one of the most common and serious neurobehavioral disorders of childhood, affecting children from early childhood into adult life. Over the 16 year period, stimulants, primarily methylphenidate hydrochloride (Ritalin), came to be used exclusively in the treatment of A.D.D. and A.D.H.D. The editorial goes on to point out that physicians give children Ritalin for inattentiveness rather than hyperactivity. This caused a constant rise in the number of prescriptions. But inattentiveness is a completely different problem and does NOT require Ritalin.

On December 1, 1995, the *Wall Street Journal* ran a front-page story citing the case of a 10-year-old boy on 30 mg of Prozac (usual adult Prozac dosage is 20 mg per day) because psychiatrists prefer to use drugs rather than psychotherapy. Recent research suggests psychotherapy plays an important role, even in the age of wonder drugs like Prozac, Zoloft, and Paxil. Psychological upheavals affect brain chemistry, a strong vote for talk therapy. Joseph Coyle, Chairman of the Department of Psychiatry at Harvard Medical School, released this information. Many behavior therapists feel the use of Ritalin or Prozac may be covering up the real problem.

According to the *Physician's Desk Reference (PDR)*, side effects of Ritalin include headaches, insomnia, loss of appetite to anorexic behavior, stunted growth, memory loss, hostility, and even suicidal behavior. In some cases, the child becomes violent with everyone. Other reported side effects include loss of energy, a flat-look, zombie-like, sadness or depression, withdrawal, loss of taste, tics, skin rashes, muscle spasms, and psychosis. Given all this documented information regarding adverse side effects, drug sales for hyperactive/A.D.D. children are still booming. It's no surprise that the drug companies are the largest money making businesses in the world.

The *PDR* states there is neither specific evidence that clearly establishes the mechanism whereby Ritalin produces its mental and behavioral effects in children, nor conclusive evidence regarding how these effects relate to the condition of the central nervous system. It's tragic that very young hyperactive or inattentive children are sometimes placed under the care of a chemical baby-sitter or a chemical straight jacket, and not just for months but for years.

A report in *Psychopharmacology Update* February, 1996, outlined results of a double-blind study of Tegretol and reported the drug is not effective in controlling children with conduct disorder characterized by severe aggression. Jeannette Cueva, M.D., Medical Director of the Child Psychiatry inpatient unit at St. Vincent's Hospital and Medical Center in New York, found little difference between Tegretol and a placebo. Dr. Cueva reported the use of Ritalin failed to reach superiority over a placebo in a study

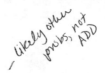

likely other probs, not ADD

of institutionalized delinquent boys aged 9 to 14.

Tricyclic antidepressants have mixed results in studies. Dr. Cueva also reported, "Overall, it appears that stimulants and tricyclic antidepressants fail to produce a satisfactory response." Dr. Cueva stated neuroleptics are the most common agents in the treatment of aggression even though it is believed that this effect is nonspecific, but the usefulness of these medications is limited by the development of adverse effects, including sedation, dystonic movement (abnormal muscle movement), withdrawal, and tardive dyskinesia (syndrome of potentially irreversible, involuntary slow movements in patients treated with neuroleptic drugs). Dr. Cueva reported the findings at the annual meeting of the American Academy of Child and Adolescent Psychiatry in New Orleans.

Dr. Diane McGuiness, Professor of Psychology at the University of South Florida, warns, "The amphetamines interact with dopamine and norepinephrine. The consequences of a prolonged use of amphetamines could produce subsequent changes in the production and action of these two neurotransmitters."

In *The Myth of the A.D.D. Child,* Dr. Armstrong noted a study that appeared in the *Journal of Psychiatry Research.* The journal reported a significantly greater frequency of cerebral atrophy (abnormalities in the brain) in young adult males who had taken stimulant drugs, like Ritalin, during childhood. The past use of drug treatment (Ritalin and other stimulants) could have been a possible cause.

Parents of children who are patients at the Pain & Stress Center reported teenagers who had been on Ritalin, had to be given tranquilizers to help them calm down, especially when these children go through the hormonal changes of puberty. One 13-year-old was given Ritalin for A.D.D., and Zoloft to help him calm down and sleep. This child is now free of all medications and is using biofeedback, counseling, and amino acids.

On January 13, 1996 the Associated Press reported that government scientists uncovered the widely used children's drug, Ritalin, might cause cancer in mice. Ritalin has been sold for 40 years, but it came on the market before drug makers were required to test for carcinogenicity. The National Toxicology Program, a branch of the *National Institute of Health,* routinely tests such older drugs for possible risks. When the FDA obtained the study, they made Ritalin's manufacturer, Ciba-Geigy Corporation, put a warning about the findings on the drug's label and notify doctors about the potential risks. *pg 13 scup only 6 mill kids have*

Recent reports demonstrate prescriptions for Ritalin are *ADD* up two and a half fold in the last five years, and if the trend continues, up to 20 million children will be on this powerful drug by the year 2005. A December 1995, report on *ABC's 20/20* noted Ritalin is being sold on the street like uppers—which is exactly what it is. Another report stated the use of Ritalin had become so prevalent that the manufacturers were fearful they would not have enough.

Stressed parents look for relief, anything to get the school off their backs. So they turn to Ritalin because they have been told, *it's a magic bullet.* An important note concerning Ritalin: physicians do not understand how it works in the brain, just that it is a stimulant that calms children down. Any stimulant will calm *ADD* children or adults down. That is how stimulants work! They suppress creative thinking, communication, or any desire to verbalize ideas and spontaneity.

Dr. Steven E. Breunig of the University of Pittsburgh Medical School, and a leading researcher on drug use with mentally retarded children, has shown that more than 20 percent of the children taking major tranquilizers or stimulant-type drugs will develop permanent tardive dyskinesia. This is a serious disorder characterized by epileptic-type movements of the mouth, arms, neck, and trunk. Dr. Breunig has also shown that the drugs can impede the child's ability to learn, cause blood disorders and eye problems, suppress appetite, cause insomnia, and generally dampen the child's emotions. One of the most frequent side effects that we hear the most about with Ritalin is that the child becomes *zombie-like.*

How Ritalin works is not fully known, but medical experts at universities conclude that Ritalin stimulates activity in parts of the brain that assist concentration and impulse control, and raises the serotonin level in the brain. As part of the limbic system in the brain it responds to the amino acids GABA, glutamine, and glycine. These amino acids therapeutically affect brain chemistry. Ritalin has no therapeutic value—it does not enhance, it suppresses! But tryptophan, an amino acid with no side effects whatsoever, raises the serotonin level of the brain naturally. Tryptophan converts to 5-HTP in the brain. This is discussed in detail in the section on amino acids.

Traditional medical treatment for hyperactivity has been, and still is, administering behavior-altering drugs like Ritalin, Cylert, Thorazine, Dexedrine, Adderall, and Mellaril. Now there are reports of Prozac, Zoloft, and Xanax being used for anxious children. Anxious children don't need drugs; they need understanding and guidance. Important note about Cylert (pemoline): if your child takes Cylert, it is very important to monitor his or her liver functions, since 2 to 3% of people taking this medication can develop chemical hepatitis.

When a child is kept on one of these controlled drugs, the cause of the anxiety or hyperactivity still remains. In short, the medication may keep a lid on the undesirable behavior of the hyperactive child, but it does absolutely nothing to solve the basic problem in the child's body and brain.

Special Note: According to the *PDR,* Ritalin should never be used in children under six years of age, since the safety and efficacy of Ritalin for this age group have not been established. Neither is sufficient data available on the safety and efficacy of long-term use of Ritalin in children. Manufacturers have not provided conclusive scientific proof that Ritalin, or any other psychotropic drug, is not harmful to children. The latest published data reveals drug manufacturers are now targeting children. Peppermint Prozac is the latest to lure parents into the drug trap. Children are being given Xanax, Zoloft, Prozac, and Effexor, just to name a few. According to Arianna Huffington, nationally syndicated columnist in *U.S. News and World Report,* August 18, 1997, "At least 580,000 children are being prescribed antidepressants—and those numbers are likely to increase dramatically."

IMS Health, a research firm that follows the prescription drug industry, reported in 1999 and 2000 more than 19 million prescriptions for various drugs were filled. For A.D.H.D. and A.D.D., this is an increase of 11 million-prescription over the previous five years. *This makes no sense*

In August 2000, *USA Today* reported some schools were accusing parents of child abuse if they would not give their children Ritalin. In this feature story, writer Karen Thomas reported that some parents gave in and medicated their child because they feared having them taken away. In many cases, Child Protective Services in the New York area has gotten involved to the point of visiting parents who take their children off Ritalin and citing medical negligence.

This type of fear enforcement has gone too far, pitting educators against parents. Many physicians and therapists feel the use of hard drugs might be covering up the real problem; children have anxiety, and if they have experienced a traumatic episode such as September 11, their behavior is impacted by their fear. The key for parents is to explore all of the possibilities, then decide a direction that gives their child a chance to live drug free.

As you will see throughout the book, the key lies in neurotransmitters, the chemical language of the brain. Using amino acids and nutrients is only putting back in the brain what belongs there.

Doctors make it too easy for parents to send their kids to Camp Prozac rather than to good counselors who help them resolve the issues they seem to find as stumbling blocks. If drugs are used to help them resolve their problems, then solutions to future problems are all just a pill away.

According to Thomas J. Moore, senior fellow in health policy at George Washington University Medical Center and author of *Prescription for Disaster: The Hidden Dangers in Your Medicine Cabinet,* prescription drugs cause 100,000 deaths annually, more than twice the number of auto accidents.[7] In a recent issue of the *Journal of the American Medical Association (JAMA),* Dr. Bruce Pomeranz states that over two million patients are hospitalized ... gravely ill from adverse reactions to drugs. No figures are available on the number of patients that consult a physician for drug reactions, but do not need hospitalization.

Drug reactions are the sixth leading cause of death in the U.S. The risk of a serious side effect from prescription drugs is 26%, or 26 out of 100. Compared to the risk of a serious auto accident at 2%, the risk of a serious reaction to a medication is 12 times more likely than a serious auto accident. According to Dr. Pomeranz, even with serious reactions to over-the-counter or prescription drugs, 1 in 15 hospital patients, or 5%, die from these reactions. Thomas Moore concludes that prescription medications, "rank as one of the greatest man-made dangers in modern society." Prescription medications are "a major peril to public health." One of the most hazardous activities of modern society is taking prescription medications.

Ritalin is now prescribed to almost 10% of all male children to control their behavior. Yet Ritalin's mode of action is not completely understood. Ritalin often produces side effects such as insomnia, appetite loss, tics, twitching, Tourette's syndrome (a form of brain damage), abnormal sounds or movement, stunted growth, and stomachaches.

Stimulant Medication Side Effects

Common initial side effects (try dose reduction)
- Anorexia
- Weight Loss
- Irritability
- Abdominal pain
- Headaches
- Emotional oversensitivity
- Easy crying

Less Common Side Effects
- Insomnia
- Dysphoria or exaggerated feelings of depression and unrest without apparent cause (especially at higher doses)
- Decreased social interest
- Impaired cognitive test performance (especially at higher doses)
- Less than expected weight gain
- Rebound overactivity and irritability (as dose wears off)
- Anxiety
- Nervous habits (such as picking at skin, hair, etc.)
- Withdrawal effects
- Insomnia
- Rebound attention deficit hyperactivity disorder (ADHD)
- Depression (rare)
- Hypersensitivity rash, conjunctivitis or hives

Rare but potentially serious side effects
- Motor tics
- Tourette's disorder
- Depression
- Growth retardation
- Tachycardia
- Hypertension
- Psychosis with hallucinations
- Stereotyped activities or compulsions

Side Effects reported with Cylert (pemoline) only
- Choreiform movements (nervous condition marked by involuntary muscular twitching)
- Dyskinesias (defect in voluntary movements)
- Night terrors
- Lip licking or biting
- Chemical hepatitis (elevated liver enzymes, jaundice, epigastric pains)

But the long-term effects are unknown. In *Prescription for Disaster*, Moore quotes the manufacturer of Ritalin, "Sufficient data on the safety and efficacy of long-term use of Ritalin are not yet available."

Clinical trials for most medications are only a few weeks in length, yet it is not uncommon for prescriptions to be taken for years, which is the norm for Ritalin and other medications used for hyperactivity or A.D.D. Drug companies do not usually evaluate drugs for long-term effects. *Are the drug companies really looking out for your safety?* The pharmaceutical industry spends more than $10 billion a year to convince you (and your physician) to buy more prescription drugs.

If God had intended Ritalin or other prescription drugs to be in our brain, he would have put it there in the beginning.

Hyperactivity/A.D.D.
Or Allergic Reactions

In 1988, when I wrote the first edition of *Control Hyperactivity,* I briefly mentioned food allergies and chemical sensitivities as a cause of hyperactivity and A.D.D. Since that time, I have had the opportunity to consult with Dr. Doris Rapp, one of the world's foremost authorities in environmental medicine.

Environmental illness (E.I.) is the name for an assortment of medical problems that can affect almost any area of the body. Dr. Rapp states, "One of the most distressing problems caused by E.I. is brain allergies, or brain fog." The E.I. patient cannot think clearly, remember, or learn at the level needed. Dr. Rapp outlines, in detail, the causes of E.I. and effective treatment in her best selling book, *Is This Your Child's World?* For the many years of dedication and contributions in the field of environmental medicine, I feel Dr. Rapp certainly deserves a Nobel prize. Through her books, tapes, lectures, and numerous personal consults, I have come to realize that thousands of children are misdiagnosed every year because their physicians are not aware of what the real problem is or could be. Before a prescription for Ritalin or any other drug is given, physicians should look at what Dr. Rapp refers to as *The Big Five.* The Big Five systematically pinpoints the specific causes of E.I.

Repeated scientific studies indicate that food allergies cause as many as sixty-six percent of A.D.H.D. children's symptoms. I encourage parents to ask their pediatrician to read Dr. Rapp's book. The book is a wealth of information that took years of research to compile.

The Big Five

1. Symptom, behavior, and memory

How does the child feel, behave, and think before, during, and after school?

2. Appearance

How does the child look?

Do they have red earlobes, dark circles under the eyes, or a runny nose?

Does the child have wiggly legs?

Does the child constantly clear his throat or do the nasal salute (wiping his nose in an upward direction)?

3. Writing or drawing

Are there changes in how the child writes or draws before and after eating certain foods, or after exposure to chemicals via touch, smell, or ingestion (i.e., pesticides on fruit or vegetables)?

4. Breathing

Does the child develop asthma, or breathing problems, after being exposed to chemicals or foods?

5. Pulse

Does the child's pulse increase by more than 20 beats after eating, or after exposure to an offending substance? A normal pulse ranges between 65 to 80 beats per minute. If a child's pulse increases suddenly while resting, it may be due to an offending substance causing an allergic reaction.

Source: *Is This Your Child's World?* by Doris Rapp, M.D.

Unrecognized Sensitivities to Food, Dust, Mold, Pollens, or Chemicals

The following list comprises behavioral indications of children who may have unrecognized sensitivities to food, dust, molds, pollens, or chemicals.

- Learns well one day (or hour), but the next day (or hour) he cannot. *yes*
- Appears unable to learn or behave most of the time. *No*
- Suffers from recurrent headaches, leg aches, muscle spasms, or constant digestive *yes* complaints and bedwetting.
- Seems unable to consistently function well in school. *?*
- Displays behavior and personality changes. *yes – who is it*
- Is too active or too tired. *sometimes* *who doesn't*
- Has congestion or asthma. *sometimes*

If these illnesses and problems can be recognized in the early stages, children avoid the many emotional, learning, and health problems that interfere with their ability to reach full potential. If any of these symptoms describe your child, then you should consider blood tests to help you adjust his diet and environment as soon as possible. The blood test provides an effective means of revealing the offending foods. In many cases, the foods eaten on a regular basis cause numerous problems and are known as hidden food sensitivities. The blood test uncovers hidden sensitivities and confirms the foods that cause immediate or delayed food reactions.

Most parents never suspect that their children's, or their own, medical or emotional complaints could be due to an environmental illness. Even with a multitude of warning signs along the way, many parents do not pay any attention until notes start coming home from school, or the child is in the second or third grade and doing poorly.

Parents should be aware of the following behavior patterns if they occur at an early age. If your baby falls out of the crib, walks at eight months, and has chronic ear infections, breathing problems, congestion, or skin rashes, these symptoms should lead you to a possible allergy connection. Be aware of toddlers who have constant temper tantrums, are very sensitive to loud noises, or have a constant runny nose, leg pains, stomach aches, and gas. By the time these children start school they cannot sit still. They display irritability, aggressiveness, biting, and they punch and kick parents, as well as other children. They may cough when they laugh, run, or exercise. Their symptoms intensify when they are exposed to cold air and cold drinks. On damp days, they may start wheezing as though they are developing asthma.

Children with E.I. become fatigued, withdrawn, irritable, and will pull away if you try to touch them. A reaction can cause children to cringe and hide in a dark corner. Some children become depressed and even suicidal after eating certain foods or when exposed to pollens, molds, dust, or chemical odors. Many have short fuses and will explode with anger and rage for no apparent reason. They fear rejection and withdraw from relationships.

Handwriting is a sure way to follow the hyperactive child's behavior—they may go from large to small dots, neat and readable to illegible. Certain children develop characteristic symptoms when they have a reaction.

Symptoms include:

- Puffy bags or wrinkles under the eyes
- Dark blue, black, or red eye circles
- Red ears
- Nose rubbing
- Wiggly legs
- Spaced-out look

These signs reflect the behavioral patterns of allergic-tension-fatigue syndrome.

Other *typical allergic reactions* include:

- Asthma
- Hay fever
- Eczema or hives
- Muscle aches and spasms
- Headaches
- Leg aches
- Irritability
- Fatigue
- Depression
- Belligerence
- Temper tantrum
- Disturbed sleep
- Bed-wetting
- Digestive upset
- Learning difficulties

Some children do not have typical allergic responses. They may display only the latter symptoms or complaints not usually recognized by allergists and physicians as being related to allergies.

Many of these varying clusters of problems are, indeed, caused by an allergic reaction to different foods, chemicals, dust, pollen, and molds. Dr. Rapp believes allergies can strike anywhere on or in the body, and affect emotional stability. She does not limit allergy symptoms to hives, hay fever, and asthma. Some children also demonstrate numerous wild mood swings, as well as the inability to learn for the same reason(s).

Dr. Rapp's views are shared by thousands of physicians and therapists who practice environmental and orthomolecular medicine. They are convinced that many behavioral, emotional, and physical problems not conventionally accepted as allergies can readily be caused by sensitivity to different factors in the environment or diet.

Many doctors think allergies affect 10 to 15 percent of the population. But researchers have demonstrated this problem as much more pervasive. In some schools an estimated 25 percent of children take Ritalin. If you ask teachers who have been teaching for twenty or thirty years, they will tell you there is no comparison to how children were before and how they are now. "The problems don't end with childhood," says Dr. Rapp. "The disease inside little bodies continues and you eventually have an irritable, repressed, and fatigued adult, who doesn't live up to his or her potential, can't form a good relationship with the opposite sex, or can't hold a job." This predisposes a person to a lifetime of mind-altering drugs.

Dr. Rapp questions how many general practitioners, psychiatrists, pediatricians, neurologists, psychologists, teachers, or parents are not aware that foods, pollens, molds, dust mites, pets, and chemical pollution are clearly environmental factors. Any of these can cause some children to become hyperactive, inattentive, and impulsive. If environmental factors are not considered, many children can be needlessly placed on Ritalin or other mind-altering drugs. Allergy sources can be found everywhere—home, school, inside, or out. Children can be sensitive to a pet, a carpet-cleaning chemical, or the synthetic carpet itself, to mouthwash, to the toothpaste with red dye and sugar, or to the teacher's perfume. All are possibilities.

According to Dr. Markus J. Kruesi, Chief of Child and Adolescent Psychiatry at the Institute for Juvenile Research, "What we are all beginning to conclude is that bad environments that more and more children are being exposed to are, indeed, creating an epidemic of violence. Environmental events are really causing molecular changes in the brain that makes people more impulsive." Ronald Kotulak published Dr. Kruesi's research in *Inside the Brain*. Other studies in this text confirm children with low serotonin levels have problems with behavior disorders, as well as aggression and depression.

In many school districts, the use of ventilation systems is reduced to cut heating or cooling bills. The result: poor air circulation which affects sensitive children who may then react to chemicals and disinfectants in the bathrooms, on the desktops, the floors, in the gym, or in the cafeteria. Children can become limp or even hyperactive from the sprays used on their desks in the classroom. When the children go outside, instead of fresh air, they may encounter air laden with pesticides, fungicides, or herbicides. A sensitive youngster can enter a lavatory, encounter a barrage of odors and chemicals, and exit in an altered state, unable to write or concentrate in class. If your child demonstrates unusual behavior, or complains of headaches or nausea, go to the school as parents should do, and literally see, smell, and touch your child's environment. Walk into the gym. Do you smell fresh floor wax? You may have to visit the principal and request a moratorium on floor wax for a couple of weeks, and see if there are any changes. In cooperation with school authorities, some parents have installed air purifiers to clean the air in their children's classrooms. The purifier helps remove dust, molds, and chemicals. Affected children often improve. Entire classrooms often experience fewer infections.

Once you figure out the cause of the problems, you can do something about them. But if you don't take the time, no one else will. Research and read as much you can on the allergy-behavior connection, and, if possible, take the affected child to a specialist in environmental medicine. These practitioners help parents remove the nails from the shoe and don't just put ointment on the sore. They teach parents how to recognize and remove the causes of their children's illness, instead of treating the symptoms with drugs.

Educated parents should no longer feel helpless or guilty. You quickly learn to recognize why your child suddenly becomes ill or acts inappropriately. After changes are made in the diet, at home or school, you can make the decisions that promote long-term wellness rather than chronic illness within the family.

According to Charles Gant, M.D., Ph.D., an orthomolecular specialist in Syracuse, N.Y., "Psychotropic drugs for kids are absolutely obsolete." Dr. Gant recently completed a study demonstrating that A.D.D. and A.D.H.D. patients on nutritional therapies achieved similar behavior improvements as patients on Ritalin.

Dr. Gant's patients have shown a 95 percent success rate using nutritional supplements. He believes nutritional supplements work because it's what we are made of. Dr. Gant conducts several lab tests to establish imbalances—then he prescribes a complete nutritional program using amino acids, essential fatty acids, vitamins and minerals. The goal is to establish what the problem is and correct it so that the child will continue to improve.

The following are medical symptoms that are due to allergic reactions that you might observe in your child. Dr. Rapp refers to this as the *allergic-tension-fatigue syndrome*.

Medical Symptoms of Allergic–Tension–Fatigue Syndrome

Nose	Year-round stuffiness or congestion, mucus-filled or watery nose, sneezing, nose rubbing.
Aches	Head, back, neck, muscles, joints, growing pains or aches unrelated to exercise, stiffness, swelling.
Belly problems	Belly aches, nausea, upset stomach, bloating, bad breath, gas, belching, vomiting, diarrhea, and constipation.
Bladder problems	Wetting pants in the daytime or in bed, constant need or rush to urinate, burning or pain with urination.
Face	Pale, dark eye circles; puffiness or wrinkles under the eyes.
Glands	Swelling of lymph nodes in the neck.
Ear problems	Repeated formation of fluid behind eardrums, ringing ears, dizziness, excessive perspiration, and low-grade fever.
Mental	Inability to focus on one project, constantly moving hands or feet; headaches, neck and shoulder pain.

Dr. Rapp reports some children suffer from fatigue, tiredness, weakness, mental confusion, irritability, drowsiness, depression, body aches, fever, chills, and night sweats. These children often sleep poorly, awaken at night, have nightmares, and cry out in their sleep. Often these children experience learning problems.

Using this information as a guideline, watch your child's behavior for one week, to see what he does, and how he acts in specific situations. At the same time, add to your log what he eats—especially how much sugar and caffeine he consumes.

Physical Symptoms of Allergies

Tension headaches

Itchy, watery eyes

Red eyeballs

Anal itch

Fluid behind the
   eardrum

Ringing in the ears

Hearing loss

Red, rosy cheeks

Red earlobes

Dark circles under the
   eyes

Wrinkles under the
   eyes

Cracks at the corners
   of the mouth

Hoarseness

Rapid heartbeats

Heart palpitations

Belching

Heartburn

Indigestion

Stomachaches

Spastic colon

Diarrhea

Hives

Eczema

Muscle cramps

Backaches

Frequency and burning
   with urination

Anemia

Sluggishness

Depression

Restlessness

Nervousness

Tremors

Emotional outbursts

Destructive behavior

Anxiety, fear

Phobias, panic attacks

Spacey feeling

Memory loss

Inability to concentrate

Irritable behavior after
   meals

Food Allergy Screening

Recent interest in the food allergy problem has risen from growing recognition in medical literature. Estimates indicate about sixty percent of the U.S. population suffers some form of food allergy. These food allergies can cause or complicate a health problem. Adverse food allergy symptoms prove extraordinarily diverse.

Food reactions encompass two major types: immediate and delayed.

Immediate Food Reactions

Food reactions occurring within three hours after eating are called immediate. Generally, high IgE antibody levels present in the blood cause the reaction. IgE antibodies produce immediate allergic reactions and are the "classic" allergy reaction with which many people are familiar. Obvious reactions can include rash or headaches after eating or drinking an offending food.

Delayed Food Reactions

A delayed food reaction usually occurs hours or up to three days after consuming the offending food. Sometimes if you eat a food for several days (e.g., not going a day or two without eating it), you could develop a reaction to it. Delayed reactions are more difficult to recognize, and are most often called hidden food allergies.

The immune response to delayed food reactions is more complex and less defined than the immediate type reaction. In most cases, delayed reactions involve other antibodies such as IgG, IgM, and IgA. These antibodies combine with food particles in the blood, forming complexes that cause inflammatory reactions in the tissues.

Allergic Conditions

An allergic condition suggests something is wrong biochemically, such as faulty absorption of food, a depressed immune system, Candida yeast infection, weakened adrenal glands, or a lack of needed nutrients.

Effect of Food Additives

Ben F. Feingold, M.D., of San Francisco, wrote a book in 1975 entitled *Why Your Child Is Hyperactive.* This book quickly caught on throughout the nation. Dr. Feingold believes hyperactivity is mainly due to artificial food colorings, artificial flavors, and natural salicylates. Though he notes that some children are also affected by other items such as dust, pets, pollens, and odors, he does not believe that allergies directly relate to hyperactivity. Dr. Feingold is quick to point out that Ritalin and Cylert, the most commonly prescribed medications for hyperactivity, contain artificial colorings. All food additives must be considered potential allergic or toxic troublemakers for the hyperactive child.

In some cases, a child may have an allergic reaction to a specific chemical additive; again, the total load of the chemical additives contained in the child's diet and his medication may produce a toxic effect. If a certain food is definitely implicated as an unwanted cause of hyperactivity or A.D.D. behavior, eliminate it from the child's diet for at least three months.

The food elimination diet provides an excellent way to find out what foods cause allergies in your child. Two-time Nobel Prize Laureate, Dr. Linus Pauling, says a child must follow a dietary regime not deficient in the essential nutrients. This echoes the principle that "you are what you eat,"—and what you don't eat.

The late Dr. Carl Pfeiffer, noted orthomolecular physician

and past director of the Brain Bio-Center, po
one of the major underlying causes of hyp
children is a chemical imbalance in the child's biochemistry.
The imbalance could be serotonin, the most widespread
neurotransmitter system in the brain. Serotonin affects
the regulation of the limbic system, cortex, cerebellum,
basal ganglia, and hypothalamus. Dr. Pfeiffer feels parents
should first remove sugar, food additives, and caffeine
from children's diets. Then, for proper neurotransmitter
function, address amino acid and nutrient deficiencies.

Dr. Jeffrey Bland, a leading scientist in nutritional
medicine states, "There is an exciting new development
in the field of neuropharmacology that for the first time,
(... recognizes that) diet may have an impact on brain
neurochemistry; amino acids can actually influence
regulatory substances that may ultimately and clinically
cause changes in mood, mind, memory, and behavior."

Serotonin is the *Master Controller!*

Signs of Serotonin Deficiency

- Depression
- Anxiety/Panic Attacks
- Migraine Headaches
- PMS
- Carbohydrate/sugar cravings
- Insomnia
- Obesity
- Fibromyalgia
- Alcoholism
- OCD (Obsessive-Compulsive Disorder)
- Aggressive or violent tendencies
- Chronic Pain
- Hyperactivity

Sugar Addiction

In Dr. Janice Phelps' book, *The Hidden Addiction and How to Get Free,* she states sugar addiction causes many insidious symptoms not recognized right away. Children can have extreme reactions to sugar, such as aggressive behavior, excessive movement, and hyper speech. When withdrawn from sugar and provided with complex carbohydrates and the proper amino acids, vitamins, minerals, and protein, children demonstrate marked improvements.

Dr. Phelps reports sugar addiction is the world's most widespread addiction, and the hardest one to break. *Sugar addiction* refers to both refined sugar and simple carbohydrates. Complex carbohydrates break down more slowly, so they enter the system more slowly and do not invoke hyperactive symptoms, as do simple carbohydrates.

Sugar addiction is so widespread and is shared by so many addictive children, as well as adults, that Dr. Phelps identifies it as the "basic addiction" preceding all others. Sugar dysmetabolism is a major factor in the profile for addiction. Sugar addiction can last a lifetime, or the sugar addict may progress to other addictive substances such as alcohol, street drugs, or prescription drugs.

Most addictive people suffer other symptoms as a direct result of their disturbed carbohydrate metabolism. Children addicted to sugar go through mood swings—false highs and lows. Sugar predisposes them to possible addictive behavior. Research studies demonstrate the amino acid, glycine, can be used successfully to help break a sugar addiction. Glycine has a calming effect and is an inhibitory neurotransmitter in the brain. A documented example: a nine-year-old boy had a craving for sweets every day after

fructose? simple carbs in it simple carb

school. With orthomolecular therapy he was given a 250-mg capsule of pure glycine by sprinkling it on a half piece of fruit, or on an oat-bran muffin, or ¼ teaspoon of glycine powder was added to his fruit juice. His mother reported he was completely satisfied and the craving decreased.

Gymnema Sylvestre, a herb from India, proves very effective as a sugar blocker. Gymnema aids in controlling sugar cravings and the uptake of sugar into the bloodstream, and is effective for both children and adults. Gymnema also helps maintain normal glucose levels.

Recently, at the Pain and Stress Center, I saw a girl named Julie—an 11-year-old whose parents were concerned about her behavior. Her teacher told them she was hyperactive and suggested Julie be put on Ritalin. I asked her parents to take all sugar products out of her diet, and as they eliminated them, write down the product name and how much sweetener was included (that information is usually on the side of the box.) The next time I saw Julie, her mother and I figured out she was consuming in the range of 20 to 25 teaspoons of sugar per day. A dietary evaluation

Food	*Sugar Content*
12 ounces soda drink	12 teaspoons
12 ounces chocolate malt shake	18 teaspoons
1 cake donut	4 teaspoons
1 cup vanilla ice cream	7 teaspoons
1 piece apple pie	15 teaspoons
1 cup sugar-coated cereal	8 teaspoons
1 white flour waffle, plain	5 teaspoons
1 chocolate éclair	10 teaspoons

and a complete blood study on Julie revealed high triglycerides and cholesterol—especially for an eleven-year-old child. Julie was placed on an orthomolecular supplement program and scheduled for behavioral modification therapy.

After three weeks the difference was almost unbelievable. Julie was happy and smiling, and sat quietly reading a book while I spoke with her mother. In one month Julie was a different child—happy, smiling, and well-behaved. Julie's mother heard other parents talk about their children's behavior changes when they were placed on Ritalin. She also heard about all the adverse side effects, in addition to it being extremely addictive. She was so right!

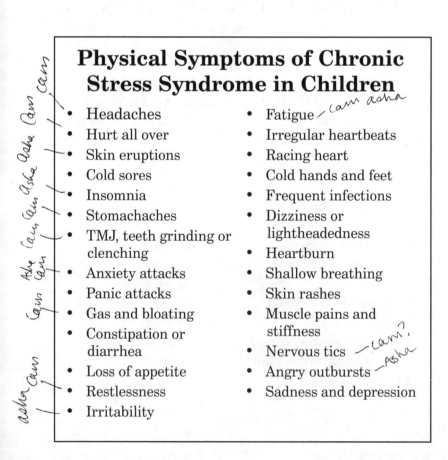

Physical Symptoms of Chronic Stress Syndrome in Children

- Headaches
- Hurt all over
- Skin eruptions
- Cold sores
- Insomnia
- Stomachaches
- TMJ, teeth grinding or clenching
- Anxiety attacks
- Panic attacks
- Gas and bloating
- Constipation or diarrhea
- Loss of appetite
- Restlessness
- Irritability

- Fatigue
- Irregular heartbeats
- Racing heart
- Cold hands and feet
- Frequent infections
- Dizziness or lightheadedness
- Heartburn
- Shallow breathing
- Skin rashes
- Muscle pains and stiffness
- Nervous tics
- Angry outbursts
- Sadness and depression

As mentioned earlier, not only is Ritalin addictive, but it falls in the category of a Schedule II drug, in the same class with morphine and opium. Yet doctors prescribe Ritalin for our children without a second thought.

Julie did not need Ritalin. She needed a healthy diet and specific nutrients in her brain to establish her molecular balance.

Sugar Health Briefs . . .

A constant sugar craving is a direct indication that you have an addiction, and the sugar is at work destroying your body.

Sugar addiction causes headaches, joint pains, gas gains, bloating, and fatigue. If these symptoms are part of your problem, you must begin to decrease sugar intake as soon as possible.

Sugar can cause food allergies, endocrine problems, hypoglycemia, diabetes, tooth decay, osteoporosis, arthritis, cancer, and many other degenerative diseases.

When you eat sugar continously, your body becomes inefficient at manufacturing glucose from complex carbohydrates, proteins, and fats.

Researchers have found that eating sugar increases the excretion of calcium. When you eat sugar your blood calcium increases, and you excrete it. You are pulling the calcium from the bones and tissues where it is stored.

Homeostasis is a wonderful balance in the body. It involves a constant fine tuning of the body chemistry.

Behavior Characteristics And Brain Chemistry

The hyperactive A.D.D. child displays a multitude of behavior characteristics. Most of these reflect the inability of the central nervous system to effectively modulate motor activity.

A significant fact about hyperactivity is that it really affects less than thirty percent of the individuals with attention deficit disorder. We find this extremely interesting, since for many years everyone with attention deficit syndrome was referred to as hyperactive. Hyperactivity ranges from minor fidgeting, or finger tapping, to the more overt behavior of hyperkinesis, when the child is in perpetual motion from dawn to dark. Hyperactive children usually have restless sleep cycles and short sleep patterns. A low serotonin level affects the sleep pattern.

Mary Coleman, M.D., Ph.D., conducted a study and found all hyperactive children have low serotonin levels. A proper combination of tryptophan or 5-HTP and B6, elevates the serotonin level and balances the brain; the child's symptoms diminish. The dosage, of course, depends on the child's age, weight, and the degree of hyperactivity. As stated before, when you correct nutrient deficiencies and feed the brain properly, the child's behavior changes accordingly.

One of the behaviors most often mistaken for A.D.D. is chronic anxiety. Children can display both aggressive and passive behavior. They cling to their parents and fear any new situations, or constantly argue. Part of the hyperactive A.D.D. child's behavior includes low self-esteem, frustration, and dependency. Children want help and do not understand why they behave the way they do. If they take Ritalin, they become more withdrawn and will not verbalize their feelings. Young children don't know how to say, "Please help." But they will say, "Please don't make me take Ritalin anymore."

These were the words of a little boy named Scott in 1984, when his mother brought him to my office to evaluate his aggressive behavior. The question in my mind was, "why Ritalin, a powerful stimulant." My search began for the proper nutrients that affect brain chemistry, and would help children without harming them. Scott's problem was specific amino acid deficiencies, and allergic reactions to what his mother thought was the best thing she could give him—milk. His mother eliminated milk from Scott's diet, and his behavior improved remarkably.

Many professionals in the mental health field use the DSM V (Diagnostic Criteria Manual). The DSM established the guidelines for universally accepted diagnoses.

The DSM V lists the following as Attention Deficit With Hyperactivity (A.D.H.D.).

A. *Inattention.* (Child must demonstrate at least 3.)

1. Often fails to finish thing he or she starts.

2. Often does not seem to listen.

3. Easily distracted.

4. Has difficulty concentrating on schoolwork or other tasks requiring sustained attention.

5. Has difficulty sticking to a play activity.

B. *Impulsivity.* (Child must demonstrate at least 3.)

1. Often acts before thinking.

2. Shifts excessively from one activity to another.

3. Has difficulty organizing work.

4. Needs a lot of supervision.

sometimes

5. Frequently calls out in class.

X6. Difficulty awaiting turn in games or group situations.

C. *Hyperactivity.* (Child must demonstrate at least 2.)

sometimes

1. Excessively runs about or climbs on things.
2. Has difficulty sitting still or fidgets excessively.
3. Has difficulty staying seated.
4. Moves about excessively during sleep.
5. Is always "on the go" or acts as if "driven by a motor."

For Attention Deficit Without Hyperactivity (A.D.D.), the criteria are the same as above except the child never has symptoms of hyperactivity (criterion C).

In the same DSM under Generalized Anxiety Disorder, you will find at least half of the symptoms listed. The symptoms include hyperattentiveness, difficulty in concentrating, irritability, and impatience. Could it be that many of these children have anxiety for valid reasons and are not A.D.D. or A.D.H.D.? My own research and patient interviews certainly support this theory.

Parents and educators, as well as the general public, have been brain washed to think of A.D.D. or A.D.H.D. as some type of mental illness. Physicians, especially those in pediatrics, endorse the mental illness aspect because it supports the drug therapy. Parents are pushed and shoved into believing their children have a mental problem. So, why not drugs?

Dr. Russell Barkley, a psychologist and advocate of Ritalin and other drugs, feels there is something wrong with these children. On December 10, 1995, Dr. Barkley appeared on a *60 Minutes* investigative report of Ritalin abuse. Dr. Barkley stated, "What's wrong in people with A.D.H.D. is a serious failure in the brain's inhibitory system, the ability of the brain to inhibit and control itself." Dr. Barkley referred to Ritalin as brake linings of the brain that are being energized, and that's why Ritalin works so well for A.D.H.D. children. It does not make them more active; it makes them more focused, more subdued, more inhibited!

Dr. Barkley did not completely explain brain function and Ritalin activity. What Dr. Barkley did not say was this: the part of the brain that controls inhibition, emotion, and memory is part of the limbic system in the brain, specifically, the amygdala. The limbic system comprises the amygdala and hippocampus, which are connected to each other forming a circuit that strongly influences the regulation of emotions and is the storehouse of emotions. The limbic system's multiple connections to the frontal lobe affect the area of the brain involved with speech and coordination of feelings and perceptions. Research demonstrates that alterations of function in the limbic system can cause such changes in emotional response as rage, calm, anger, anxiety, fear, memory, and attention. ← memory & attention are emotional responses

James Swanson, a Professor of Pediatrics and an expert in A.D.H.D., stated on *60 Minutes,* December 10, 1996, "Nationwide, the number of kids (… on Ritalin) is staggering." Dr. Swanson reported approximately 2 million children were diagnosed and treated in 1994. In 1990 and 1991, there were 1 million. So the figures continue to double. He noted many children with A.D.H.D. are not helped by medication.

Dr. Swanson stated there is no foolproof test for A.D.H.D. So many of the new cases are misdiagnosed. He felt 25 to 30 percent of the diagnosed children may not actually have the disorder. Lesley Stahl, on *60 Minutes,* reported that, "Hundreds of thousands of American school children are being diagnosed and medicated by mistake." Ms. Stahl reported, "Not only are kids misdiagnosed, they are given medicine when they don't have the disorder."

The pharmaceutical industry markets drugs through the media to establish the problem as a chemical imbalance in the brain. Dr. David Kaiser reported in his article, "Psychiatry Betraying and Drugging Children," this is absolutely not true. In 1996, he stated, "Modern psychiatry has yet to convincingly prove the genetic/biological cause of any single mental illness." Peter Breggin, M.D., in his best selling book, *Brain Disabling Treatments in Psychiatry*, states, "At present, there are no known biochemical imbalances in the brain of typical psychiatric patients—until they are given psychiatric drugs." In other words, Breggin believes no chemical imbalances exist until you take psychiatric drugs. When the media successfully secure the cooperation of unwitting parents, it establishes a dangerous precedent.

Military Rejects Ritalin Users

With the use of Ritalin at an all time high and spiraling out of control, parents are forced with a new dilemma—military rejection. All branches of the armed forces reject potential enlistees who have used Ritalin or other drugs that change or modify behavior. The defense department has a long-standing directive instructing recruiters to reject those men and women who took Ritalin for academic problems. Even though the drug is no longer taken, it is considered a mind-altering drug. The military feels Ritalin users pose a risk because they needed the medication to succeed in school. Basic training now involves a lot of classroom work. Parents, physicians, and teachers are unaware the military services are exempt from the Americans with Disabilities Act and can discriminate against young people who have used behavior modifying drugs, especially Ritalin.

Cox News Service, "Using Ritalin makes many unable to enlist in military," *San Antonio Express News,* November 28, 1996, p. 20A.

Children and their parents actually begin to believe they have something wrong with their brains, and they feel they can't learn without Ritalin or another psychiatric drug.

Ritalin's manufacturer admits it is a drug of dependency, another way of saying that it is a drug of addiction. Dr. Breggin also spells out the damage done to a child's brain and future problems that can exist when they take Ritalin. The documentation is there; children treated with a stimulant will suffer from multiple drug-induced biochemical imbalances. Ritalin and other stimulants cause major changes in the vital neurotransmitter system of the brain and decrease the over all flow of blood to the brain.

Thomas Armstrong, Ph.D., psychologist, wrote *The Myth of the A.D.D. Child,* a text that provides parents fifty innovative, proven, and safe ways to help children develop lifelong internal controls. Dr. Armstrong, in an interview on *CNN,* November 2, 1995, stated that some children get labeled A.D.D. and the problem may be stress or even a different learning style. Some children may have food allergies or a chemical imbalance, but neither is a reason to use powerful stimulant drugs such as Ritalin. Dr. Armstrong feels teachers and physicians have gone haywire diagnosing children as A.D.D. and then immediately turning to the use of Ritalin.

Recently Prozac, Zoloft, Paxil, and Effexor have been added to the list of drugs given to children with A.D.D./A.D.H.D. Prozac, Zoloft, Paxil, and Effexor have stimulant effects such as hyperarousal, anxiety, and panic in the brain. But, drugs are what psychiatrists understand best, not talk therapy or brain deficiencies. With fear and anxiety already a problem for misdiagnosed A.D.D. children, increased drug use could cause multiple problems, including phobias.

Where will it end? When will it end? When you, the parents, who brought them into the world, take a stand and say NO. *NO DRUGS FOR MY CHILD!*

Stimulant Effects on the Brain

According to Peter Breggin, M.D. in his best selling book, *Talking Back to Ritalin,* he states Ritalin and other brain stimulants create severe biochemical imbalances. Stimulants do not *normalize the brain;* they render it abnormal. Stimulants produce pathological malfunctions in the child's brain.

Dr. Breggin is an expert in the negative effects of drug therapy such as Ritalin. Dr. Breggin maintains that stimulants and amphetamines have an extremely negative impact on the brain—by reducing overall blood flow, disturbing glucose metabolism, and possibly causing permanent shrinkage or atrophy of the brain. Ritalin as well as other stimulants produce a loss of various neurotransmitters that can become permanent. Stimulants can also act as false neurotransmitters changing the chemistry of the brain with irregular flow. Stimulants and amphetamines can impair the limbic system, the region of the brain that regulates and conveys emotion and mood to the cerebral cortex. The cortex controls intelligence, concentration, and problem solving.

From ages four to ten new learning and experiences are reorganized and reinforced through connections between brain cells. As a child learns new things, new connections form, and neuron development enhances. Ritalin and other stimulants can interrupt blood flow and connections between brain cells. Stimulants can make some children more active, and others more withdrawn and despondent. Stimulants can worsen pre-existing tic disorders in children who have a risk for the disorder. A major problem in both children and adults using stimulant medications is Tourette's Syndrome.

Orthomolecular Therapy

The controversy will continue for years to come. Pediatricians will tell parents not to worry. "Just feed your child a well-balanced diet, and he will get everything he needs."

Simply feeding a high-quality diet to A.D.D./A.D.H.D. hyperactive children cannot equate to high-quality and optimal nutrition. Many complex factors affect digestion, absorption, and even the transportation of food (that could be faulty). Optimum nutritional benefits depend on a multitude of factors; everything must function smoothly from the time the first bite is taken until the nutrient reaches the body's cells. If an imbalance occurs due to improper bodily functions, then you will experience an excess or deficiency of some kind. If the imbalance continues, a minor problem can develop into a major disease.

Our food today does not have the nutritional value we need. Polluted air, antibiotics, chemicals, and insecticides—all toxic and harmful—contaminate the foods. Fast foods have now entered the schools along with candy, cookies, and soft drinks, most of which contain high contents of sugar and caffeine. How can you possibly feed your child a perfectly well balanced diet, as pediatricians tell you to do, if the nutrient value of the food has less than 50 percent of the needed nutrients.

The U.S. Agricultural Department states that food is colored to make it "look good." But the nutritional value in food is low or does not exist. American people believe the fallacy that if they consume certain numbers of calories in specific food groups, their dietary needs will be met. This, of course, should include the proper number of vitamins, amino acids, and minerals. But instead of being in an optimally nourished state, we find suboptimally nourished children. The state of their nutrition is the state of their health. Further, the absence of disease does not necessarily mean the presence of wellness.

So, why should our children be exempt from proper nutrition? Nutritional deficiency disorders can and do occur, and in our own country we see malnutrition by over consumption and under nutrition. This simply means we eat too much of too little.

If a child has food allergies and their nutritional intake is restricted, diet becomes an even bigger problem, along with absorption. This is a major problem, not only with hyperactive and A.D.D./A.D.H.D. children, but also for adults with high stress and active lifestyles.

Amino Acids and Neurotransmitters

Diet alone cannot supply *ADD?* children with optimum levels of nutrients needed by their unique biochemical and nutritional conditions. Amino acids are used for A.D.D. and A.D.H.D. behaviors to restore the disturbed biochemical homeostasis causing impaired functions in the child's brain. The amino acids literally feed the brain and restore the balance that nature intended.

Amino acids are the building blocks of proteins in the body. We cannot live without these proteins. Our children were not born with Ritalin in their brain. So, how can they have a Ritalin deficiency? Neurotransmitters underlie every thought and emotion, memory and learning; they carry the signals between all nerves or neurons in the brain.

A stimulated brain cell releases a neurotransmitter that carries a message to the next cell. The neurotransmitter fills the cell, causing that cell to be stimulated. Then another message is released. All this happens in the brain in a split second, allowing the message to travel quickly from one cell to the next, along neuropathways. Thousands of these pathways carry messages to specialized areas of the brain.

This means all messages come in at once with equal velocity. The A.D.D. child's brain functions like a telephone switching station at Christmas when everyone tries to call at once. All he gets are busy signals, and the messages do not reach the proper receptor site.

Neurotransmitters have the responsibility for behavior and learning. Consequently, a neurotransmitter deficiency has a dramatic effect on children's or adults' abilities to learn and function in an orderly manner. Most hyperactive and A.D.D. children are born with a shortage of neurotransmitters, which tends to run in families, mainly on the male side. Hyperactive A.D.D./A.D.H.D. children do not manufacture the needed extra neurotransmitters. Drugs do not create neurotransmitters; *they use only what is there.*

Where do we get neurotransmitters? Neurotransmitters come from the amino acids such as GABA, glycine, taurine, tyrosine, glutamine and tryptophan. Do children or adults get enough aminos through diet? NO! Balanced aminoacid doses, in the right combination and formulas, produce the needed neurotransmitters naturally. Using a stimulant medication to try to produce them is like a shotgun gun going off in the child's brain.

Approximately fifty different neurotransmitters exist in the human brain, but communication between brain cells uses only ten (approximately) major neurotransmitters. Certain neurotransmitters carry pain sensations, while others order voluntary muscle movement; some cause excitatory emotional responses; others are inhibitory. The neurotransmitters that govern our excitatory emotional responses are called catecholamines, noradrenaline (norepinephrine), and adrenaline (epinephrine). All three derive from the amino acids, phenylalanine and tyrosine.

Our reactions to everything we encounter, the way we are stirred by a song or an old picture, angered by an argument or emotional pain inflicted by someone we love, or amused by something we see on television—all these emotions depend on the chemical language of the brain, specifically, neurotransmitters. Too much, or too little, of any of these substances will make us under or overreact according to the stimulus.

How we feed the brain directly affects our production of neurotransmitters. Neurotransmitters determine our mental and emotional state of well-being. Accordingly, with proper nutrition and supplementation, we can correct or enhance mind, mood, memory, and behavior.

All major neurotransmitters are made from amino acids and from dietary protein. One of the dangers of a low-protein diet is not ingesting enough amino acids to make adequate brain neurotransmitters. Apathy, lethargy, difficulty concentrating, loss of interest, and insomnia all result when your diet includes low amounts of amino acids. A.D.D. and hyperactive children, as well as adults, have low levels of neurotransmitters. When drugs are used, the drugs do not produce or increase production of neurotransmitters. *Drugs only address symptoms.*

At the Pain & Stress Center over the past 20 years, we've seen major successes when using a specialized amino-acid program. The results are happy, healthy children, who are drug free. Amino acids restore the balance nature intended.

A neurotransmitter is the chemical messenger or language sent between brain cells. Chemical messengers transmit thoughts from one cell to another, allowing brain cells to talk to each other. In order for the brain to be chemically balanced, all the major neurotransmitters and neuropeptides must be present and available in ample amounts. An insufficient level of neurotransmitters can upset the balance of the brain chemistry.

Can you how to how much?

Nerve Cells and Neurotransmitters

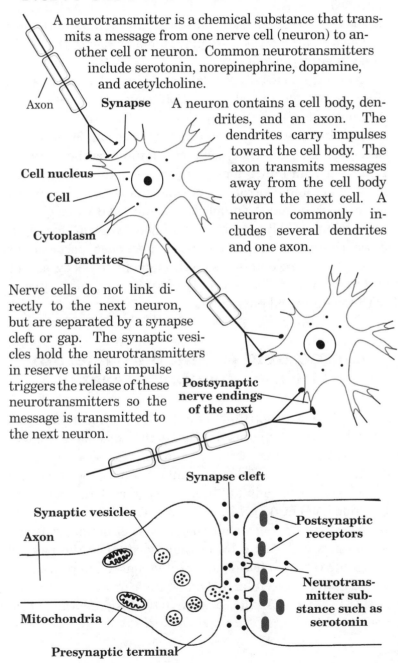

A neurotransmitter is a chemical substance that transmits a message from one nerve cell (neuron) to another cell or neuron. Common neurotransmitters include serotonin, norepinephrine, dopamine, and acetylcholine.

Axon   **Synapse**   A neuron contains a cell body, dendrites, and an axon. The dendrites carry impulses toward the cell body. The axon transmits messages away from the cell body toward the next cell. A neuron commonly includes several dendrites and one axon.

Cell nucleus

Cell

Cytoplasm

Dendrites

Nerve cells do not link directly to the next neuron, but are separated by a synapse cleft or gap. The synaptic vesicles hold the neurotransmitters in reserve until an impulse triggers the release of these neurotransmitters so the message is transmitted to the next neuron.

Postsynaptic nerve endings of the next

Synapse cleft

Synaptic vesicles

Axon

Postsynaptic receptors

Neurotransmitter substance such as serotonin

Mitochondria

Presynaptic terminal

Some of the major symptoms of neurotransmitter deficiencies are A.D.D., A.D.H.D., brain fog, mood swings, increased stress, anxiety, depression, insomnia, irritability, and aggression. Stress also plays a major role in the depletion of neurotransmitters.

Neurotransmitters regulate mind, mood, and behavior. Researchers have established that neurotransmitters and neuropeptides are the keys to behavior, emotions, and pain. Scientists have identified more than 50 different neurotransmitters that conduct communication between brain cells, but only ten play major roles. Inhibitory amino acids affect and control this chemical language. Inhibitory amino acids include tryptophan, taurine, GABA, and glycine. For example, GABA, an inhibitory neurotransmitter, slows down the anxiety-related messages between parts of the brain. GABA receptors reside throughout the body, as well as in the brain. That's why GABA has a calming effect—both mentally and physically.

Amino Acid & Nutrient Therapy (Orthomolecular Therapy)

The Pain & Stress Center uses the following amino acids, vitamins, and minerals in the orthomolecular program for A.D.D./A.D.H.D. children and adults. The program outlined includes specific amounts of amino acids needed by the child's (or adult's) brain to correct deficiencies and to reduce A.D.D./A.D.H.D. behavior. The shotgun approach is never used; giving a child mega doses of amino acids and vitamins will do more harm than good. For the past 20 years our research has demonstrated marked improvement in children using a total orthomolecular program to control A.D.D. behavior. All the children in the program were drug-free.

Symptoms of Amino Acid Deficiencies

- ADD/ADHD
- Alcoholism
- Ammonia toxicity
- Anxiety
- Arthritis
- Ataxia (defective muscular coordination)
- Behavioral disorders
- Blood sugar imbalances
- Cardiovascular disease
- Chemical intolerances
- Chronic fatigue
- Chronic gastrointestinal distress or bowel irregularity
- Depression
- Dermatitis (inflammation of the skin)
- Detoxification impairments
- Excessive inflammation
- Failure to thrive (infancy)
- Family history or early symptoms of degenerative disease
- Frequent headaches or pain
- Frequent colds, infections, and persistent inflammatory responses
- Hyperlipidemias (high blood lipid levels)
- Hypertension (high blood pressure)
- Hypotonia (loss of muscle tone)
- Hyperactivity
- Inflammatory disorders
- Impaired mental development
- Insomnia
- Intolerances (persistent) to foods and chemicals
- Mental problems
- Mental retardation
- Mood swings
- Myopathies (muscular diseases)
- Neurological disorders
- Neural tube defects (birth defects)
- OCD (Obsessive Compulsive Disorder)
- Ocular (eye) disorders
- Osteoporosis
- Oxidative stress
- PMS
- Poor immunity
- Poor wound healing
- Recurrent ear infections
- Rheumatoid arthritis
- Seizures
- Short stature or chronically underweight, growth failure (children)
- Weak skin and nails

Source: Diagnostic Value of Amino Acid Analysis, Great Smokies Diagnostic Laboratory, 2000

TRYPTOPHAN

Tryptophan, an essential amino acid necessary to maintain the protein balance in the body, plays a variety of important roles in mental activity. The serotonin neurotransmitter in the brain helps control moods. To have enough serotonin you need enough tryptophan or 5-HTP, which is essential to serotonin's formation. B6 (pyridoxine) or P5'P (pyridoxal 5'phosphate) is needed to form serotonin. P5'P is the biological form of B6 and is nontoxic. Many A.D.D./A.D.H.D. children have low serotonin, tryptophan, and B6 levels. Tryptophan raises low levels of blood serotonin. Supplements containing tryptophan and B6 sometimes correct some of the biochemical disorders related to aggression.

Studies done at the North-Nassau Mental Health Center in Mannasett, New York, reports sufferers of obsessive-compulsive behavior demonstrated signs of improvement following treatment with tryptophan and B6. An article published by the *American College of Nutrition* in June 1987, showed specific doses of tryptophan and other amino acids can replace Ritalin and Cylert, without the adverse side effects.

Tryptophan brings up the serotonin level gently and normally. Tryptophan or 5-HTP doses should be based on the level of a child's A.D.D./A.D.H.D. No two children are alike—they are all biochemically unique, and should be addressed (treated) accordingly. Orthomolecular therapy provides positive results and, in most cases, dramatically reduces hyperactive behavior. The child demonstrates, among other qualities, a willingness to cooperate with his parents and teachers. We've seen these changes in a majority of children who have previously failed to improve with the use of powerful stimulant drugs or tranquilizers. The major-

why expensive? [handwritten note]

ity of children seen at the Pain & Stress Center have been exposed to many forms of drug treatment—all with little or no success—that include Ritalin, Cylert, multiple tranquilizers, and sedatives.

5-HTP (5-Hydroxytryptophan)

Cam Asha [handwritten note]

5-HTP offers needed help for those suffering from anxiety, depression, sleep disorders, hyperactivity, chronic stress syndrome, PMS, obsessive/compulsive behavior, addiction, and constant carbohydrate craving. 5-HTP or 5-Hydroxy-l-tryptophan is a natural extract from the Griffonia plant seed. Griffonia acts by providing the body with 5-HTP, or 5-Hydroxytryptophan, an amino acid that easily crosses the blood-brain barrier, and converts into serotonin as a natural process.

Serotonin is one of a dozen brain neurotransmitters responsible for communication between the cells. Without neurotransmitters you would not be able to think, function, or even live. The brain, spinal cord, and intestinal tract contain the serotonin receptor sites.

5-HTP is safe and effective. 5-HTP is free from side effects and has no reported toxicity or contraindications. Researchers observed a definite link between depression, addiction, obsessive/compulsive behavior, and serotonin deficiency. Serotonin plays a key role in numerous brain functions—as the level of serotonin decreases, maladaptive behavior increases. The serotonin system represents the largest single neurotransmitter system in the brain, influencing multiple functions such as moods, movement, behavior, and eating patterns. 5-HTP from the Griffonia seed is being established as a true solution to those who need more serotonin.

In the body, tryptophan converts to 5-HTP, which then converts to serotonin. Serotonin undergoes additional conversions in the pineal gland to yield melatonin that is responsible for inducing sleep. Serotonin is the brain's master impulse controller for all emotions and drives. Symptoms of aggression and anger develop when your serotonin level is low. Aggression is one of the most widely recognized signs of low serotonin in the brain. Addictive and compulsive behavior, headaches, pain, and depression are warning signals that your brain needs more serotonin.

Millions of people have turned to SSRIs (Selective Serotonin Reuptake Inhibitors). SSRI drugs such as Prozac, Paxil, Zoloft, and Effexor work by selective enhancement of serotonin levels. SSRIs prevent the presynaptic nerve from reabsorbing serotonin that it previously secreted. By inhibiting the normal process, Prozac causes an increase in brain serotonin levels; but Prozac and other prescription drugs do not increase neurotransmitters. Decreased serotonin levels in the brain are also associated with obesity and alcoholism. A low serotonin level causes the brain to send signals of hunger or craving. Many antidepressants cause the brain to rev up, causing a false euphoria, mood swings, as well as aggressive behavior.

In *Vitamin Research News,* March 1998, Dr. Ward Dean was asked, "Can you use 5-HTP with Prozac?" Dr. Dean answered, "Yes, you can (and probably should) use 5-HTP with Prozac. However, you will probably have to reduce your dosage of Prozac after starting 5-HTP in order to prevent a serotonin excess syndrome."

Prozac increases the amount of serotonin in the synaptic clefts between nerve endings, but does not do anything to replace the tryptophan required for the body to manufacture serotonin. Consequently, many Prozac users become deficient in tryptophan, resulting in increased requirements for Prozac which just makes the situation worse. Many former users of Prozac were able to completely discontinue their antidepressants by replacing them with 5-HTP; but this should be done with the help of a physician or qualified health care professional. 5-HTP elevates the serotonin level of the brain naturally, without side effects or drug dependency.

5-HTP is synergistic with other supplements that enhance neurotransmitters. These supplements include the amino acids GABA, glutamine, tyrosine, DLPA, and glycine. Magnesium prolongs the benefits of 5-HTP, especially magnesium chloride found in Mag Link. Chronic stress syndrome will deplete available serotonin, as well as interfere with serotonin's ability to control behavior. Research has demonstrated a low serotonin level can change brain function and impair learning.

Children with low serotonin levels demonstrate abnormal carbohydrate metabolism, causing low levels of blood sugar and defective nourishment to the brain. The key to the improvement of a hyperactive or A.D.D. child is a balance of neurotransmitters, the chemical language of the brain. Smooth brain functioning requires biochemical homeostasis. As mentioned earlier, homeostasis can be disturbed by food allergies or other medical problems. The importance of a healthy, well-nourished, efficiently functioning brain cannot be overstated.

The brain is the busiest, yet the most undernourished organ in the body. Proper nourishment for your child's brain directly affects his or her production of neurotransmitters. Neurotransmitters determine mental and emotional states of well-being.

Scientists now believe low serotonin may be responsible for an increase in depression and drug use among teens and children. Most teens with low serotonin levels are more prone to try recreational drugs or even prescription drugs for relief. A low brain serotonin level impairs the ability to focus and reason. 5-HTP shows a lot of promise as a natural answer to a multitude of problems that plague adults and children.

5-HTP can be found in combination formulas for children. These include HTP10 Complex and Teen Link. Consider your child's particular problem(s), and select the formulas that best address his problem. Take caution with children. Adjust doses according to age, weight, and the particular problem. If prescription medication is being taken, use extreme caution with 5-HTP. The two in combination could cause problems such as "serotonin syndrome." Serotonin syndrome causes symptoms of irrational euphoria, diarrhea, agitation, confusion, and gastrointestinal upset. If you are taking Prozac, Zoloft, Paxil, and Effexor, do not combine them with 5-HTP unless your physician, or qualified health care professional, directs you to do so.

GABA (Gamma Amino Butyric Acid)

GABA, an inhibitory neurotransmitter, is found through-out the central nervous system. GABA assumes an ever-en-larging role as a significant influence on A.D.D., A.D.H.D., stress, anxiety, and depression, as well as stress-induced ill-nesses. By 1998 there were over 3,000 documents, articles, and texts on GABA, and how it affects stress/anxiety in the brain. According to Candace Pert, a neuroscientist who discovered the GABA receptor, every cell in the body has a GABA receptor—one reason why GABA has such positive effects.

If you examine a step-by-step process of what happens in the brain when a child feels stress and anxiety, you can see how GABA works to slow down messages. Panic, anxiety, or stress-related messages start to release numerous signals. Simultaneously, a physiological response begins to take place—the fight-or-flight syndrome.

The unceasing alert signals from the limbic system eventually overwhelm the cortex (the decision-making part of the brain), so the cortex and the rest of the brain's stress network become exhausted. The balance between the limbic system and the rest of the brain to communicate in an orderly manner depends critically on inhibition. GABA inhibits the cells from firing, diminishing the anxiety-related messages from reaching the cortex.

GABA fills certain receptor sites in the brain and body. This slows down and blocks the excitatory levels of the brain cells waiting to receive the anxiety-related, incoming message. When the cortex receives the message, it does not overwhelm the child with anxiety. He is able to maintain control and remain calm. But, when under prolonged stress or anxiety, the brain exhausts all the available GABA and other inhibitory neurotransmitters, thus allowing anxiety to attack from every direction. His ability to reason diminishes. In a full-blown anxiety or panic attack, physical symptoms include excessive sweating, trembling, muscle tension, weakness, loss of control, disorientation, difficulty breathing, constant fear, headaches, diarrhea, depression, and unsteady legs.

Tranquilizers provide only temporary relief. We have seen many patients on Xanax that still experience anxiety. They have been told it is not addictive—it is! *THERE IS NO SUCH THING AS A TRANQUILIZER DEFICIENCY!* Nutrient deficiencies do occur, however; they can and do change behavior. Human behavior involves the functioning of the whole nervous system, and the nervous system requires amino acids. GABA, glutamine, and glycine prove vital for energy and the smooth running of brain functions.

B6 (pyridoxine) is GABA's most important partner. We have successfully used GABA, glutamine, and glycine with patients to ease anxiety, irritability, and A.D.D.

Research demonstrates a large number of children who display A.D.D./A.D.H.D. behavior are, in fact, experiencing anxiety that is interpreted as A.D.D. If they use all available GABA, then the receptors in the brain become empty, allowing the brain to be bombarded with random firings of excitatory messages. These receptor sites in the brain, when filled with appropriate amounts of GABA, prevent the reception of multiple random firings so the brain does not become overwhelmed. In *Lancet*, August 14, 1982, a research report regarding tranquilizers and GABA transmission clearly stated, GABA is a major inhibitory neurotransmitter in the mammalian central nervous system and the nutrients that raise the brain's GABA concentration possess a sedative anticonvulsant property.

At the Pain & Stress Center we regularly combine GABA and other amino acids to achieve positive results. Dose amounts vary, depending on the age and weight of the child. We consider the child's levels of stress and anxiety, his diet, and his overall behavior. The combination of GABA, glutamine, glycine and other specific nutrients has proven successful with A.D.D. and A.D.H.D. children.

An A.D.D. child's limbic system (the emotional part of the brain) stores anxiety and stress. Under prolonged periods of stress, the limbic system releases the anxiety-related messages to fire at the cortex, or the "thinking part" of the brain; the child becomes overwhelmed, and the result includes either hyper-aggressive or hyper-passive behavior. The child totally loses control and displays irrational behavior.

GABA now takes its place as a major influence on those taking drugs, in many cases replacing the drugs. We have found that, when combined with other amino acids, GABA works exceptionally well with A.D.D. children, both aggressive and passive.

CAUTION: DO NOT buy just any GABA and mega dose your child. *Too much GABA, as with anything, can cause problems and side effects.*

L-GLUTAMINE

This amazing amino acid, along with GABA and Glycine, is rapidly becoming the most important therapeutic amino acid of the twenty-first century. Glutamine, found in many foods, is the third most abundant amino acid in the blood and brain. Glutamine provides a major alternative fuel source for the brain when blood sugar levels are low.

Glutamine functions as an inhibitory neurotransmitter and is the precursor for GABA, the antianxiety amino acid. Glutamine helps the brain dispose of waste ammonia, a protein breakdown by-product which irritates brain cells, even at low levels. Recent scientific research regarding glutamine demonstrates its link to the most important functions of the body's vital organs and musculoskeletal system. Glutamine aids the body in muscle development when illness causes muscle wasting. Muscle wasting occurs following a high fever, chronic stress, illness, or a traumatic accident.

The amino acid trio of Glutamine, GABA, Glycine, and the B6 cofactor represent the major inhibitory neurotransmitters in the brain. Glutamine is found in the nerves of the hippocampus, the memory center of the brain, in the cranial nerves, and in many other areas of the brain. These three amino acids work together as inhibitory neurotransmitters, the chemical language of the brain. Anyone taking amino acids must take B6 to metabolize the amino acids.

Glutamine studies reported intellectually impaired children and adults demonstrated an increase in IQ after taking glutamine in combination with ginkgo and B6. Research done by Dr. Roger Williams, at the University of Texas, Clayton Foundation, demonstrated children and adults classified A.D.H.D. showed a marked improvement when taking glutamine, 250 mg to 1,000 mg daily. Dosage depended on age and weight.

At the Pain & Stress Center we use a Balanced Neurotransmitter Complex (BNC) plus GABA powder or Super BNC capsules, along with glutamine and Huperzine. Our results have been excellent. The Balanced Neurotransmitter Complex formula assists brain communication, allowing the brain cells to talk to each other.

Recent discoveries have shown 50 or 60 neuropeptides can be found in the immune system as well as the brain. Each unique neuropeptide has its own receptor. These intercellular neuropeptides and receptors mediate communication among the brain, glands, and immune system. A neuropeptide is a peptide comprised of amino acids that are the building blocks of proteins. Neuropeptides and their receptors are the biochemical correlates of emotion.

GABA and glutamine are not only found in the brain, but also in the receptor cites throughout the body. Amino acids can and do enhance mind, mood, memory, and behavior. A particular herb, Huperzine, shows excellent results in enhancing concentration. Huperzine increases blood flow to the head, improves mental functioning and the ability to focus for longer periods of time.

Glutamine is known as the M & C amino acid, memory and concentration. Seventy five percent of hyperactive and A.D.D. children's blood tests (serum plasma) showed low levels of glutamine.

Dr. C. Frederick noticed a definite increase in the IQs of children given glutamine. When glutamine was given daily, children showed impressive improvements in their abilities to learn, to retain, and to recall. Adding glutamine in supplement form represents a major part of my orthomolecular program for hyperactive and A.D.H.D. children. Glutamine is one of the amino acids that create the needed neurotransmitters in the brain that enhance learning and memory. When tested, hyperactive and A.D.D. children showed low neurotransmitter levels, especially glutamine. Adding glutamine can increase the level of neurotransmitters. Start with 500 mg of glutamine and gradually increase until you reach the optimal dose for your child. The dosage depends on your child's weight, activity, and concentration (mg) level. The total maximum recommended glutamine dosage is 3,000 mg per day.

Research shows that glutamine protects bacteria cells

weird

against poisoning by alcohol; and in experimentation on laboratory volunteers, it stopped their craving for alcohol. This characteristic has been studied carefully. Compared with the effects of other amino acids, glutamine consistently decreases alcohol consumption.

The brain must be nourished to function properly. Whatever the brain tells the body to do, the body does. Everything starts with the brain and ends in the brain. As mentioned before, the amino acids, tryptophan (5-HTP), tyrosine, and GABA can alter the composition and the function of the brain. These amino acids function as precursors in the brain, and ultimately affect everyone's behavior.

The most exciting area of amino acid research is the study of brain metabolism. Amino acid therapies are making a great impact on general medicine, and in the field of psychiatry.

Dr. Phyllis Bronson, an expert in nutritional biochemistry and orthomolecular therapy at the Aspen Clinic, states that specific amino acids are necessary for proper neurological functioning. Subtle deficiencies of these can affect mental and emotional stability. Supplementation of specific amino acids prove useful in treating hyperactivity, depression, anxiety, headaches, PMS, mental confusion, poor memory, and concentration.

Amino acids serve as an important anti-inflammatory substance that helps control sensitivity reactions and the body's natural response system. Many children and adults with food allergies report improved tolerance of food with amino acid supplementation.

Dr. William Walsh is an authority on the diagnosis and treatment of biochemical imbalances that result in behavioral disorders, including violent behavior. He has developed a treatment program, with the late Dr. Carl Pfeiffer, to control chemical imbalances. The program consists of administering carefully controlled combinations of vitamins, minerals, and amino acids. His results have been overwhelmingly positive.

Does Dr. Walsh advocate Ritalin? No. Is Ritalin the answer? No. Does Dr. Rapp, the world's foremost authority in pediatric allergy and immunology, advocate Ritalin? No. Would I give Ritalin to my child? No!

TAURINE

Taurine is now classified as a conditionally essential amino acid in the adult; but in infants and children, taurine is an essential amino acid. As one of the sulfur amino acids in the adult, taurine synthesizes from cysteine and methionine, provided B6 and zinc are present. Taurine is found abundantly throughout the body in the heart muscle, olfactory bulb, central nervous system, and brain—hippocampus and pineal gland. Taurine participates in a multitude of functions in the body, involving the gallbladder, brain, heart, eyes, and vascular systems.

As an inhibitory neurotransmitter, taurine, after GABA, is the second-most important inhibitory transmitter in the brain. Taurine's inhibitory action in the brain equals that of GABA and glycine. Its inhibitory effect is one source of taurine's anticonvulsant and antianxiety properties. Normal central nervous system (CNS) and brain development in infants and children require taurine. Taurine protects and stabilizes the brain's fragile cell membranes. Taurine appears to be most critical during development of the CNS and muscles. Taurine also effectively controls hyperactive or hyperkinetic movements, and aids in controlling tics or other spastic conditions.

Taurine proves effective in the treatment of epilepsy, acting as an anticonvulsant. For those with epilepsy, their amino acid levels are lower than normal in over half the necessary amino acids. But the levels of taurine are higher than normal, except in the cerebrospinal fluid. Usual dosage for epilepsy is 3,000 mg per day in an adult, with a non-protein meal; in children the dose ranges from 500 to 1000 mg daily, divided.

Research shows taurine's important influence on blood sugar levels, similar to insulin's action in the body. Some children with Down's syndrome have shown an increase in IQ levels when taurine was added to their diet along with glutamine, B6, and Vitamin E. Taurine is present in high concentrations in the eye, and deficient children could have problems with depth perception. Diminished vision may be an early warning sign of the need for taurine supplementation.

A deficiency of taurine shows up in some patients with depression. A deficiency can add to chemical sensitivities and decrease the body's ability to detoxify chemicals.

The need for taurine increases whenever you experience more stress than usual, or have an illness. Formation of one of the bile acids and proper functioning of the gallbladder require taurine. The bile may be a route of excretion of chemicals detoxified by the body. Taurine is sometimes called upon to help control inflammation or infection.

Inborn errors of taurine metabolism demonstrated by children include sleep and mood disorders, constant fatigue, and an inability to gain weight.

TYROSINE ~stress depression

Tyrosine is the amino acid and inhibitory neurotransmitter that helps overcome depression. Clinical studies show that tyrosine controls medication-resistant depression.

In 1980, in the *American Journal of Psychiatry*, a study by Dr. Alan Gelenberg of the Department of Psychiatry at Harvard Medical School, discussed the role of tyrosine in the control of anxiety and depression. Dr. Gelenberg postulated the lack of available tyrosine results in deficiency of the hormone norepinephrine at a specific location in the brain, which, in turn, relates to mood problems such as depression. Children given tyrosine supplementation demonstrated a marked improvement in mental performance and mood stability.

Tyrosine, because of its role in assisting the body to cope physiologically with stress and building the body's natural store of adrenaline, deserves to be called *the stress amino acid*. Stress exhaustion requires tyrosine, which converts to dopamine, norepinephrine, and epinephrine (adrenaline).

Conversion of Tyrosine in the Liver

Tyrosine → Dopamine → Norepinephrine → Epinephrine

During periods of stress, in order to continue coping with stress physiologically, the brain requires tyrosine. We use tyrosine at the Pain & Stress Center to aid children and young teens, as well as adults, with recurrent depression and mood disorders.

GLYCINE

Glycine is a nonessential amino acid, with the simplest structure of all the amino acids resembling glucose (blood sugar) and glycogen (excess sugar converted in the liver for storage). Glycine is sweet to the taste, can be used as a sweetener, and can mask bitterness and saltiness. Pure glycine dissolves readily in water. As the third major inhibitory neurotransmitter in the brain, glycine readily passes the blood-brain barrier. The body needs glycine for the formation of DNA, collagen, phospholipids, and for the release of energy.

Studies by the late Carl Pfeiffer, M.D., Ph.D., demonstrated glycine as an important factor in psychiatric disorders. Dr. Pfeiffer's findings indicate that when glycine was administered to psychiatric patients suffering from manic-depression, even those previously unresponsive to drugs achieved major improvements.

According to Ronald Kotulak's book, *Inside the Brain,* glycine "helps trigger brain cells to fire electric charges and speed learning." Glycine helps control spasticity and seizures, and is involved in behaviors related to convulsions and retinal function.

Glycine is an essential intermediate in the metabolism of protein, peptides, and bile salts. Glutathione, a liver-detoxifying compound, must have glycine present for its formation. Glycine removes heavy metals, such as lead, from the body. Glycine decreases the craving for sugar, and, in many cases, can replace sugar on foods such as cereal. Glycine calms aggression in both children and adults. When combined with GABA and glutamine, glycine influences brain function by slowing down anxiety-related messages from the limbic system.

As a very nontoxic amino acid, both children and adults can use glycine. Glycine can be mixed with other amino acids. Doses for a child range between 500 to 2,000 mg daily, divided. Glycine exists in high concentrations in meats and wheat germ.

MAGNESIUM

Hyperactive or A.D.D. children almost always show deficiencies in magnesium. Magnesium proves necessary for proper brain energy and is the first mineral depleted when anyone—child or adult—is under stress. Magnesium is a stress mineral, and deficiency can lead to hyperactive or ADD behavior.

Sherry Rogers, M.D., an expert in magnesium research, describes in her book, *Tired or Toxic,* the physical and mental symptoms of magnesium deficiency. Dr. Rogers establishes how magnesium has a quieting effect on the central nervous system. Dr. Rogers notes both children and adults who have apprehensiveness, irritability, confusion, noise sensitivity, constant eye twitching, nervousness, tremors, muscle spasms, jerking muscles, back and neck pain, some anxiety, and fatigue, have a magnesium deficiency. We have observed this in both adults and children with A.D.D./ A.D.H.D. hyperactivity and anxiety.

Magnesium plays a significant role in sugar metabolism and in the proper utilization of carbohydrates to create energy rather than fats. Magnesium is so very important in your child's diet, especially if he displays hyperactive behavior, A.D.D., or other behavioral problems. Magnesium can be taken in liquid form, tablet, or capsule. The dose will depend on the child's weight, build, stress level, and possible allergies, both food or airborne.

A magnesium deficiency causes mast cells to release too much histamine into the bloodstream. Histamine is the culprit responsible for much of the hay fever and allergy misery experienced by so many people. At the Pain & Stress Center, we use magnesium chloride in the form of Mag Link, if a child can swallow capsules. The magnesium chloride form of magnesium is tolerated, absorbed, and more readily available to the body than any other form of magnesium. The Mag Link capsules are enteric coated so they pass through the stomach into the small intestine where absorption takes place. If a child cannot swallow the capsules, use magnesium chloride liquid, Mag Chlor 85, that can be mixed with fruit juice and given orally.

When added to the A.D.D./A.D.H.D. diet, calming effects sometimes occur immediately. Most magnesium exists inside the cells where it activates enzymes necessary for the metabolism of carbohydrates and amino acids. Magnesium helps utilize the B complex vitamins, along with Vitamin C and E. Magnesium also plays a role in the regulation of body temperature.

In 1988, a study published in *Alternative Medicine Review* (Volume 3, Number 2), linked the development of A.D.H.D. to low blood-serum magnesium levels. A group of children followed for six months were given 200 mg of magnesium a day. Researchers noted a remarkable decrease in hyperactivity in the children.

Magnesium chloride has been used in the protocol for A.D.D./A.D.H.D. at the Pain & Stress Center since 1990, with very positive results. As a major nutrient needed by A.D.D./A.D.H.D. children and adults, magnesium is the number one stress mineral needed in the body. Magnesium is responsible for over three hundred enzyme functions. Magnesium cannot be stored, and it must be taken daily. Symptoms of magnesium deficiency include asthma, migraines, eye twitches, anxiety, confusion, muscle spasms, irritability, depression, nervousness, fatigue, mood swings, PMS, hypertension, and insomnia.

CALCIUM

A calcium deficiency can induce A.D.D./A.D.H.D. behavior. A child deficient in calcium may exhibit irritability, sleep disturbances, anger, and inattentiveness. The first signs of a calcium deficiency include nervous stomach, cramps, tingling in the arms and legs, and painful joints. Calcium is a strong countering agent against lead; children with inadequate calcium in their diets could possibly have a problem with lead intoxication.

Milk is an important source of calcium for growing children, providing approximately 1,200 to 1,500 milligrams per quart. Children with sensitivities to dairy products often do not receive necessary amounts of dietary calcium or tryptophan. In at least 50 percent of children we test for food sensitivities, we find a sensitivity to dairy products.

Milk, usually the number one food allergen, especially in children, must be removed from the diet. Yet, dairy products are a major food source of calcium and tryptophan. So, if the child's diet restricts all dairy products, this could lead to a major calcium deficiency. A calcium deficiency can lead to A.D.D./A.D.H.D. behavior, irritability, memory impairment, sleep disturbances, anger, nervous stomach, cramps, and tingling in the arms and legs.

Children sensitive to dairy products must receive daily calcium supplementation in capsule, chewable, or liquid form. Children up to 10 years of age need 1000 mg of calcium daily; adolescents need 1,200 to 1,500 mg daily. For those involved in sports activities, calcium supplementation is a must.

ZINC

Zinc plays an important role in the body. This mineral controls protein synthesis in every cell of the body, helps heal burns and wounds, promotes carbohydrate digestion and organ growth/development, boosts the immune system, and protects against free radicals. Zinc deficiency is a factor involved in fatigue, susceptibility to infection, decreased appetite, lack of alertness, loss of taste, and prolonged wound healing. Important constituents in the body activity involve zinc, chromium, and magnesium, as well as the hormone insulin. Insulin is essential for the regulation of blood sugar levels. Symptoms of insulin deficiency include fatigue, poor eating habits, lethargy, retarded growth, irritability, anorexia, confusion, impaired sense of taste, acne and skin problems.

In a double-blind study, zinc gluconate lozenges decreased the length of cold symptoms in patients. One report evidenced taking zinc gluconate lozenges every two hours, while awake, reduced the number of cold symptom days by one-half.

Dosage for up to 10 years of age is 10 mg daily, and thereafter 15 mg per day.

CHROMIUM

Chromium is an essential trace mineral. Highest concentrations of chromium are found in the hair, spleen, kidney, and testes. Chromium's primary function in the body activates enzymes in the metabolism of glucose and the synthesis of proteins. Chromium helps maintain normal blood sugar, cholesterol, and triglycerides. This major mineral is involved in insulin production. When a deficiency occurs, it interferes with the maintenance of healthy blood sugar levels. Some researchers report that many disorders of glucose metabolism, such as diabetes and hypoglycemia, may actually be chromium deficiencies.

Children involved in numerous sports activities should be supplementing with chromium picolinate. Exercise can increase urinary excretion of chromium and zinc. Dose range for children is 50 to 200 mcg per day, according to the U.S. National Academy of Science. Best food sources for chromium: brewers yeast, nuts, whole grains and cereals, dry beans, peanut butter, and meat.

B VITAMINS

Several years ago, Dr. Marvin Brend first found signs of Vitamin B deficiency in the psychological category with symptoms such as fear, depression, temper tantrums, anxiety, mood swings, inability to concentrate, withdrawal, listlessness, and a general feeling of being tired. Dr. Brend suggested that the weakening effects of Vitamin B deficiency occur well before a person actually displays an acute vitamin deficiency sign.

Doctors Cschamberger and Longsdale, at Cleveland Clinic, further confirmed children with behavior disorders have chronic marginal B deficiencies. Signs of deficiencies include aggressive personality changes, sleep problems, recurring bad dreams, and heightened anxiety. The researchers were able to associate these symptoms with the consumption of diets rich in *empty* calories; i.e., foods high in sugar and fat, but low in vitamins and minerals. Many snack convenience foods, today, fall into this category of empty calories.

Parents must constantly be aware how many of these high-sugar empty-calorie snacks their child consumes daily, for this helps determine the behavioral patterns. Because marginal vitamin deficiency signs and symptoms are linked to nutrient-related conditions, physicians often miss them. Many physicians receive little, if any, education in nutrition and vitamin requirements while in medical school. Consequently, they are simply not aware of the deficiency/behavioral-pattern relationship(s).

Some of the first signs of vitamin deficiencies include: intestinal problems of unknown origin, muscle pain, sleep disturbances, headaches, emotional problems, constant fatigue and lack of energy. These symptoms may significantly improve with a proper nutrient supplementation program. Conditions of emotional or mental disturbance not related to nutrient deficiencies could still require behavior therapy. But, most importantly, parents must recognize the physical and emotional signs and symptoms of vitamin deficiencies in their child and take appropriate action before those deficiencies show in a much broader range of symptoms.

A nutrient is different from a drug; a nutrient is a food substance that, in most cases, supplies either the energy or the molecular building blocks the body requires. Some nutrients, when administered in their pure form, or simply ingested in food, can act like drugs. They give rise to important changes in the chemical composition of structure in the brain. These changes can modify brain function, particularly in people with certain metabolic or neurological diseases.

PYRIDOXINE (B6)

More than almost any other single nutrient, Pyridoxine, or B6, functions as one of the most essential vitamins involved in bodily functions. This vital nutrient in your child's diet produces essential chemicals and aids in the manufacture of proteins and neurotransmitters. B6 participates in over sixty enzyme reactions involving the metabolism of amino acids and essential fatty acids.

Normal brain function and the synthesis of DNA and RNA require B6. Pyridoxine assists in the body's water balance—for both sodium and potassium—and plays a role in immune system function, antibody production, and B12 absorption.

B6 affects mental and physical well-being. As one of the greatest fighters against hyperactivity, B6 calms the hyperactive child in much the same way as Vitamin B. Vitamin B6 and tryptophan (5-HTP) supplements can correct some biochemical disorders related to aggression. Autistic children improve when supplemented with magnesium and B6. B6 is the most important vitamin for amino acid metabolism because it is the cofactor for transamine enzymes that metabolize amino acids. Riboflavin (B2) and Niacin (B3) vitamins also play an important part in amino-acid metabolism. Note: B6 or P5'P must be present for the utilization of all amino acids.

Symptoms of B6 deficiency include: irritability, fatigue, poor concentration, poor memory, inadequate sleep, depression, and mood swings.

All foods are a source of B6, but the best food sources for B6 include: brewers yeast, eggs, carrots, meat, fish, walnuts, sunflower seeds, wheat germ, and spinach.

P5'P is an alternative to B6 that can be toxic in high doses. P5'P, or Pyridoxal 5'Phospate, is the active coenzyme form of B6, or the biological form of B6. All amino acid, and protein, carbohydrate, and fat metabolism requires P5'P. At correct dosages, P5'P is non-toxic and safe for children.

VITAMIN C (ESTER C)

Vitamin C is an antioxidant necessary for tissue growth and repair, proper adrenal gland functioning, immune system and gum health, and protection against pollution of all kinds. Vitamin C plays an essential role in the treatment of hyperactivity. The most recent clinical studies in 1987 established Ester C Polyascorbate as totally neutral; it proves four times more bioavailable than ordinary Vitamin C. As a unique, complex mixture with a different molecular personality, Ester C is the most available form of Vitamin C to the tissues of the body. Ester C finds its way into your system within 20 minutes after ingesting, and 24 hours later still works long after your body excretes timed-released forms of Vitamin C.

Children, as well as adults, need Vitamin C daily. Ester C has been extremely effective in our program, and does not cause diarrhea or gastrointestinal upset as sometimes happens with regular ascorbic acid Vitamin C. Ester C has a neutral pH of 7.0.

Dr. Jeffrey Bland, nutritional biochemist and foremost authority today in nutritional therapy/medicine, recommends a range of 500 to 2000 mg of Ester C, daily, for children. Ester C is available in a pediatric dose of 250 or 500 mg. At The Pain & Stress Center, we include the Ester C in every child's program for hyperactivity. We have had excellent responses from most children using it. Ester C, given on a daily basis, is the most inexpensive nutritional insurance policy you will ever find, with positive, long-term beneficial effects on your child's health.

Symptoms of Vitamin C deficiency include: depleted immune system, hypersensitivity, fatigue, depression, poor digestion, and increased allergies.

VITAMIN E

Normal cell functions in the body absolutely require Vitamin E. We use this essential vitamin with positive results in the treatment of hyperactive children.

Wilfrid Shute, M.D., in his book *Health Preserver*, defines the versatility of Vitamin E, and establishes that hyperactive children have a deficiency of Vitamin E. Dr. Shute states he has obtained remarkable results with Vitamin E, not only with hyperactivity, but also with learning disabilities and attention deficit disorder. Dr. Shute states Vitamin E improves the child's ability to learn even with a defective or damaged sensory channel. While it does not change the basic personality of the child, Vitamin E does enhance his ability to learn, an improvement which occurs slowly but steadily.

Vitamin E helps alleviate both aggressive and passive hyperactivity. Since it is required for normal cell functioning, Dr. Shute feels it should be kept in a child's—and even in adults'—daily regimen; he recommends 400 I.U. for a child under 10.

Skin reflects our emotions and stress. A recent patient at our clinic, a 14-year-old girl, was withdrawn and anxious and had numerous skin problems. Her skin was reflecting what she could not verbalize. With daily use of 800 I.U. of Vitamin E and Anxiety Control, in three weeks her skin began to clear and her confidence improved. If a child feels different, or feels rejected from others, because she is different in some way, behavior problems can occur, especially passive hyperactivity. Certain skin conditions prove especially vulnerable to our emotions. Unresolved anxiety is the number one problem. The major conditions that result are acne, warts, hives, eczema, herpes, and psoriasis. If a child cannot express hurt, anxiety, or fear, the skin will speak volumes.

LIQUID SEROTONIN

Liquid serotonin is an excellent homeopathic formulation for acute stress, anxiety, and A.D.D. behavior. When the serotonin level in the brain is depleted from stress, anxiety, depression, hyperactivity, or A.D.D., communication in the brain, through neurotransmitters, decreases.

Serotonin is the master controller in the brain and creates vital neurotransmitters. Serotonin can be used as needed by all ages. Use 1/2 dropper for children over 50 lbs., under 50 lbs., ¼ dropper, 2 to 5 times daily.

HUPERZINE

Huperzine A is derived from a purified compound of Chinese club moss. Clinical studies confirm Huperzine enhances memory and concentration by stimulating the production of acetlcholine. Suggested dosage is one capsule twice daily for those twelve and over. Huperzine can be taken with amino acids as part of the program. Huperzine was featured in the *Journal of the American Medical Association*. Huperzine has been part of the orthomolecular program at the Pain and Stress Center over the past several years, and our results have been excellent. Huperzine has proven to be a safe and effective agent for those who need a high production of acetylcholine.

Caution: Avoid Huperzine if you have pulmonary problems, congestive heart failure, are pregnant or lactating.

L-THEANINE

L-Theanine, or L–T, is a free form amino acid found in green tea. L–T increases alpha waves in the brain that produce enhanced focus and concentration, while at the same time keeps you relaxed, less anxious, and stressed. L-T has a major role in the formation of GABA. In 1999 in the *Journal of Food Science & Technology,* a study confirms that theanine promotes the release of neurotransmitters such as dopamine and serotonin. Theanine readily crosses the blood-brain barrier, and counters the effects of caffeine.

L–T can be taken in the capsule form, or L–T can be opened and mixed with juice. It is excellent for test anxiety or mental fatigue. Children 12 years old and over, and adults, will notice how much better they feel using L–T. L-T can be taken with other amino acids such as Anxiety Control, Brain Link, or Teen Link.

PHOSPHATIDLYLSERINE

Phosphatidlyserine is phospholipid that is a component of brain cell membranes. Clinical studies demonstrate that Phosphatidlyserine improves cognitive functions including memory, learning, concentration, and vocabulary skills. Phosphatidlyserine contains soy lechitin plus three phospholipids including phosphatidylcholine, phosphatidylinositol, and phosphadylethanolamine. Children 12 years old and over, and adults can use Phosphatidlyserine.

VINPOCETINE

The herb, Vinpocetine increases cerebral functioning. Research reports that vinpocetine increases cerebral ATP (Adenosine TriPhophate) or brain cell energy, while increasing oxygen and glucose production. Vinpocetine supports memory problems and coordination through selective positive effects on brain blood circulation. Vinpocetine may be used by children 12 years and over, and adults.

Inside the Teen Brain

Teens have special needs because their brains are a work in progress. Their brain development isn't complete until they reach their twenties. Teenagers' brains, in many ways, are closer to small children's brains than adults. Neuron development is not complete. The neurons affect, not only emotional skills, but also control physical and mental abilities.

The teen diet, from a nutritional standpoint, provides zero nutrition, so they must be supplied needed neurotransmitters to allow them to make decisions, focus and concentrate. Teens who have had amino acid analyses have shown major deficiencies in serotonin, the master controller, and inhibitory neurotransmitters such as GABA, Glutamine, Tyrosine, Taurine, and 5-HTP. One of the best ways to address their daily needs is with Teen Link on a daily basis. Teen Link is a complete neurotransmitter support formula that contains serotonin enhancing 5-HTP.

The *National Institute for Health* reports that children as young as 4 can get depressed. They become withdrawn, display sleep problems, nightmares, and appear uninterested or detached. Scientists believe there is a genetic predisposition to depression. The more you interact with a depressed person, the more likely you are to display the same symptoms. Many adolescents and teens have been misdiagnosed and put on numerous psychiatric drugs, and their real problems are never understood because they were not addressed. Depression is a treatable biological disease characterized by changes in the brain chemistry. The challenge is to address the changes in the brain chemistry and establish what neurotransmitters are needed, such as dopamine, serotonin, and GABA.

Focus and Concentration

How do focus, memory, and concentration work? They work essentially through neurotransmitters, the chemical language of the brain. Neurotransmitters control the thousands of requests from the brain cells to provide information. The brain must be able to sort through all the messages and select the proper response for each of them. The brain then sends the response to the ears, eyes, heart, stomach, and muscles, until it reaches the message center of all the organs.

The brain processes two types of memory, short-and-long-term. Before the brain stores the memory, it must first be experienced in some way by the brain. As new information comes in, it flows from the senses, and the brain briefly retains the entire stimulus. Short-term memory retains information long enough for the mind to grasp it. Unless a child makes an effort to grasp the information, it remains in the short-term memory for less than a minute.

Short-term memory holds only a limited amount of information. Researchers report the short-term memory stores an average of seven to ten items. If a child needs to retain the information for more than a minute, he must repeat it. For information to be memorized, it must be heard or read at least twelve times to be processed into long-term memory for recall as needed.

Learning should never be done in a fearful situation. When fear is invoked, the brain releases stress hormones such as adrenaline. The learning situation then becomes unpleasant, blocking focus and concentration. Fearful situations can permanently alter brain function and learning. The brain requires daily nourishment for continued focus, learning, and concentration.

Ages 1 to 3. Critically important in brain development. Learning stimulus should be pleasant and continuous.

Ages 4 to 10. As new things are experienced and learned, connections in the brain are reorganized and reinforced.

Ages 11 to 15. Physical changes continue to occur. The brain now learns and stores the memories for life.

Behavior and experiences affect brain development. Proper environmental stimulation is vital. If a child uses mind-altering drugs, the influences can remain for a lifetime.

Essential Fatty Acids

The essential fatty acids (EFAs), Linoleic acid (LA) and Alpha Linolenic acid (LNA or ANA), are the major building blocks of fats. These polyunsaturated fats are essential because they cannot be manufactured in the body and must be obtained from the diet. EFAs are vital to health and their actions include: maintenance of cell membrane fluidity and stability, development and function of brain and nerve tissue, oxygen transfer and energy production, and immune functions. A report from the Surgeon General on Nutrition and Health declares that deficiencies, excesses, or imbalances in fats are involved in 70% or more of all U.S. deaths.

Our ancestors consumed diets high in both Omega-3 (plants and game) and Omega-6 fats (from seed and nuts). The balance was 4:1. The modern diet contains little Omega-3 fatty acids and no wild game, but an abundance of processed or fried foods, salad oil, and margarine. As a result, consumption of Omega-6 fatty acids is 11 times that of Omega-3 fatty acids, resulting in an imbalance.

Linoleic acid (LA) of the Omega-6 fats is found in most

plant oils (corn, safflower, canola, sunflower), nuts, seeds, and soybeans. Alpha Linolenic acid (ALA) is an Omega-3 fat and is found only in oils from cold-water fish (mackerel, sardines, anchovies, cold liver oil, and salmon) and flax oil, but canola and soybeans contain a small amount. The key lies in a balance between Omega-3 and Omega-6 fatty acids. Excesses of either fatty acid cause problems.

Omega 3 fatty acids are anti-inflammatory (allergies, asthma, arthritis, heart disease, etc.), analgesia, and immune modulating. Recently, one study found that Omega-3 was vital to mood disorder, depression, and dementia. A recent study in children with asthma that received EPA/DHA (ProDHA) supplementation for 10 months responded with less asthma symptoms. Omega-6 fatty acids such as GLA (found in borage, black current seed, and primrose oils) also reduce inflammation, alcohol and sugar consumption, and are anti-aging.

The brain is composed of sixty-percent fat, and needs adequate amounts of essential fatty acids for proper mental and neurological functioning. Essential fatty acids are vital for effective brain development in infants and children. EFAs are found in high concentrations in the brain, and aid in the transmission of nerve impulses as well as normal brain functioning. EFAs must be obtained from outside food or supplement sources since the body cannot produce them. EFAs are found in green vegetables, nuts, soy, fish, flax, vegetable oils, sesame and pumpkin seeds.

EFAs are responsible for the makeup of structures in our bodies and cells and are necessary for everyday living. According to Dr. Patricia Kane, an expert in the area of brain function and EFAs, children and teens presenting with symptoms of A.D.D. or A.D.H.D. need Omega-3 and Omega-6 oils. Dr. Kane refers to EFAs as food for the brain.

Flax meal, Vitamin E, and DHA (docosahexaenoic found in Arctic/ North Atlantic fish) are the best sources of EFAs. But a problem with fish is the amount of pesticide and mercury that is obtained from eating it. Put freshly ground flax in soups, cereal, or sprinkle on a salad. Ground flax can be added to recipes such as meatloaf, muffins, cakes, etc. Just decrease the amount of flour slightly to compensate for the flax that you add. Take Vitamin E and DHA in supplement form according to age and weight. EFAs are an important part of a total orthomolecular program for A.D.D. and A.D.H.D. children and adults.

Low levels of DHA have been linked to reduced concentration, changes in disposition, memory loss, and visual and other neurological disorders. Patients taking DHA showed a 65% improvement in dementia symptoms in a study performed at Gunma National University medical department in Japan. Another study done at Purdue University found that A.D.H.D. may be due to insufficient intake of ALA, EPA, and DHA. These researchers conclude that supplementing with fatty acids was a useful treatment for A.D.H.D.

The Neuromins for Kids is safe and easy-to-swallow. Children should begin taking it as soon as possible. Adults should use ProDHA to increase their EFA levels. ProDHA contains a high concentration of DHA enhanced with stabilizing antioxidants for freshness and contains no PCBs or heavy metals.

Special Note: Freeze fish oil or ProDHA, then take capsules immediately. The frozen capsules move on through the stomach before dissolving. This keeps the capsules from repeating and make them more easily tolerated.

Special Consideration Of Circumstances

Children and Grief

Parents sometimes face a difficult problem helping their child through the death of a loved one. Children's feelings and perceptions are often overlooked. Grief is a deeply felt human emotion, as normal as laughing, playing, crying or sleeping. Grief is a way of saying, "I miss you, and I do not understand where you are . . . or where you have gone." When you avoid a child's reaction, you magnify his fears, and replace reality with fantasy or psychological defenses.

If a child is part of the care giving of a grandparent who dies, the child could demonstrate symptoms similar to the grandparent's illness. It is not unusual for a child or adult to react this way. Physical symptoms may not be the only manifestation of grief. Behavior marked by extremes such as aggression or withdrawal can denote repressed grief. Should this occur, find a behavior therapist; explain what has happened, then take the child to see them.

Often the surviving parent gets caught up with his or her grief and makes the mistake of not addressing the child's needs. The child will begin to act out his fears, depression, anxiety, and, most of all, the uncertainty of being left alone—of being abandoned. This behavior can be interpreted as hyperactivity/A.D.D., though it simply expresses the child's frustration.

If your family has lost a loved one, take this information into consideration before someone tells you your child is A.D.D./A.D.H.D. Many times we've heard parents say, "Since his father died, I haven't been able to reach him."

A child with these behaviors needs behavior therapy. If he does not receive proper counseling, his hostility will continue to grow and come out in physical forms such as picking on other children, striking at their surviving parent, breaking things, and aggression.

A Special Note Here: Before the age of twelve, it is very difficult for a child to understand death. Taking them to funerals where people are grieving, or having them kiss the loved one "good-bye," in most cases can have a totally negative effect. We have seen many adults still haunted by the memory of having to kiss a dead person good-bye. The mental state of a child is so delicate that all these things must be taken into consideration. Let the child verbalize what he wants. Saying good-bye is part of the grieving process. They must be able to do this in their own way.

Children and Divorce

If you are in the process of, or have recently received, a divorce, your children will need time to adjust to this major transitional change in their lives. A recent study presented to the American Association for Marriage and Family Therapy, October, 1988, by the Society for Research in Adolescence, showed divorce and remarriage are hardest on children ages 9 to 15. The study was conducted with 210 families. It is important to recognize that children in this age group are struggling to establish independence, self-esteem, and sexual identity.

Parents are role models for their children, and when one is gone, a child under ten does not understand. Reassure your child that you will not go away. He also needs time to express his feelings, fears, anxiety, and guilt. He may feel he did something wrong—even that he or she was the cause of the divorce. Only by helping him understand will these feelings go away. Do not take your child for granted, thinking that he will get over it in due time. Unless you talk to your child, the only other information he gets is from other children, who are not reliable sources.

Divorce is loss and separation. The child also experiences a certain amount of grief. The reaction of the child to this loss may be similar to a loss through death—disruptive behavior, lashing out at everyone, and anger. Some parents say their child has become unmanageable since their divorce, and that his teachers complain about his behavior. Providing the child love and understanding is paramount. Ritalin is not the answer!

Preventive Measures

One essential preventive measure a parent should take even before the divorce, separation, or an impending death, is to inform school officials. By understanding the reason for a child's behavior, they can become an important support system for the child.

My own experience can serve as an example in this situation. When I was a very small child, I lost my father. I had already been through a major trauma from a burn received at 14 months of age. Now I had to cope with this loss, and I could not understood why it happened. There were three other children in the house, and my mother worked full time, so there was very little time for me to express all my many thoughts and feelings. Mother simply did not have the time—and perhaps not the awareness—to see what I was experiencing. These bewildered feelings stayed locked inside me for a long time.

Several years later, I was able to work through my feelings with the help of a counselor. When children are put into situations they have no control over, they become fearful and withdraw. Some display feelings of separation anxiety and can't focus or concentrate because of their fear and anxiety. The stress created by new situations uses all available neurotransmitters that must by replaced.

Emotional outbursts, crying spells, and anger are the first signs, followed by headaches and stomachaches.

A frequent reaction to divorce is for the child to compete with the new parent for attention of the natural parent, and the resulting conflict can cause stress and then depression. A child must be prepared when a parent remarries, and only when the youngster's acceptance is certain should the wedding take place. This procedure will ensure that the family unit remains close.

If your child is going through this type of stress, now is a perfect time to use serotonin for sleep problems, tyrosine for depression, and GABA/glutamine (such as Brain Link OR Anxiety Control) for anxiety, or in combination. This is a crucial time for both you and your child.

Never tell your children what they will need to unlearn at a later time. At a time of crisis, the whole family suffers; this calls for understanding, communication, trust, and truth between parents and children.

In times of stress, children need more neurotransmitters. The immune system is totally depleted, and they tend to turn to junk food and sweets for satisfaction. You should make sure they receive proper supplementation to help them in times of crisis.

Rx For Disease

The greatest disease of mankind is a lack of love for children, leading to children's psychological and sometimes even physical abuse. The abuse predisposes these children to a hopeless-helpless attitude, and to disease later in life. We cannot keep blaming physical poisons, or genetic defects, for every disease. We have to realize that there are poisons in our own homes that predispose us to disease by creating certain attitudes and feelings within us.

Symptoms of Grief or Loss

- Inability to concentrate
- Vague physical symptoms
- Headaches
- Upset stomach problems
- General lethargy
- Bewilderment
- Inability to focus
- Frequent distractions
- Susceptibility to anxiety and depression
- Loss of confidence
- Crying for no apparent reason
- Separation anxiety

Sleep/Nighttime Difficulties

Deviations from normal sleep patterns, strange eating habits, and allergies frequently appear together in the hyperactive/learning-disabled child. Sometimes improving the child's diet will relieve the sleep pathology. Consider halting milk ingestion to allow comfortable sleep without bedwetting. Additionally, phlegm in the nose may dry up. Sleep is a biochemical phenomenon, but emotional influences can change sleep patterns. Sleep resistance, or the inability to fall asleep in 20 minutes, is often due to a deficiency of calcium, magnesium, or manganese. A sugary dessert may make the blood sugar fall then an adrenaline release precludes sleep.

Restless sleep or constant wakefulness, often accompanied by bad dreams or terrors, usually occur as a result of falling blood sugar and adrenaline release, plus a low serotonin level. Symptoms include a pulse rate of 120, dilated pupils, and generalized perspiration. These are caused by adrenaline, not anxiety. The adrenaline makes normal dreams scary or terrifying.

Work with your child—teach them how to relax using deep breathing. Deep breathing alone can change the chemistry of the brain and causes a state of calm relaxation. The use of relaxation tapes is excellent. If needed, use a ½ dropper of Liquid Serotonin. This reduces the amount of adrenaline in the blood stream.

Important Notice

If your child is taking prescription drugs,

DO NOT JUST STOP THEM!

Withdrawal reactions can occur.

Consult your physician or a qualified health care professional for help.

Nutritional Support Program For Hyperactivity/A.D.D.

The Pain & Stress Center in San Antonio, Texas uses the following formulas for A.D.D. and A.D.H.D support. *Not ALL formulas are needed. See Focus Program on page 96.*

1. **Anxiety Control** is an inhibitory neurotransmitter formula that quiets hyperactive children. Anxiety Control can be used for daytime hyperactivity, stress, or anxiety at night to quiet the child prior to bed.

2. **Brain Link Complex** contains the amino acids that activate the neurotransmitters in the brain. Brain Link is a powder that mixes with fruit juice for rapid absorption.

3. **Super Balanced Neurotransmitter Complex (SBNC)** is a balanced combination of the essential amino acids that create neurotransmitters in the brain, and is available in capsule form. BNC + GABA is available only in powdered form.

4. **Teen Link** Complex (ages 12 and up) is an amino acid/ herbal complex for teenagers, hyperactive, and A.D.D. children. Teen Link is a special combination of 5-HTP, Tyrosine, GABA, glutamine, taurine, and B6, and is available in capsule form.

5. **HTP10 Complex** is a special combination of 5-HTP (10 mg) with glycine, GABA, glutamine, lysine, taurine, Vitamins B6 and C, magnesium, and Alpha KG. HTP10 Complex can be used for A.D.D./hyperactive children with aggressive behaviors, or in children having prob-

lems sleeping. HTP10 also reduces anxiety and fear. *Note:* Do not use 5-HTP, if you are taking SSRI meds.

6. **Super Glutamine** is a free-form amino acid found to be deficient in hyperactive and A.D.D. children. Super Glutamine contains pharmaceutical-grade glutamine that dissolves readily in liquid and is tasteless.

7. **Cal, Mag, Zinc** complex is a special synergistic combination of calcium, magnesium, and zinc for maximum absorption.

8. **Mag Link** is magnesium chloride. Magnesium chloride is the form of magnesium that is present in the body, and in capsule form is better tolerated and absorbed than any other form of magnesium. Mag Link capsules are enteric coated, and are designed to pass through the stomach and dissolve in the intestine where absorption takes place.

9. **Taurine,** a free form amino acid, is needed for proper growth and brain function. Taurine helps excessive movement, tics, or seizures.

10. **Glycine** is a free form amino acid and one of the most important neurotransmitters. Glycine can be used, without worry of adverse side effects by sprinkling on food as a substitute for sugar. Glycine assists in calming aggressive, hyperactive behavior, and is available in 250 mg capsules or in powder form. Glycine mixes readily and is sweet.

11. **NAC** is an amino acid used with bronchitis, allergies, sinusitis, and otitis media (earache). NAC is a mucus-reducing agent that decreases sinus drainage. NAC can be used even on 5-year-old-children.

12. **Gymnema Sylvestre,** an herb, helps control sugar cravings in children and adults. Children should take 1 before each meal.

13. **T-L Vite,** a one-a-day-multi-mineral vitamin capsule,

provides the body with all the basic nutrients. Calcium, magnesium, and zinc must be taken separately.

14. **5-HTP, or 5-Hydroxytryptophan,** is pharmaceutical-grade 5-HTP in capsule form. 5-HTP helps alleviate insomnia and aggressive behavior, and is available in 50 mg capsules. Use 5-HTP (50 mg), if the person weighs over 100 pounds. *Note:* Do not use 5-HTP, if you are taking SSRI meds.

15. **Liquid Serotonin** is a homeopathic formula for sleep and anxiety. Liquid Serotonin may be used as needed, and is safe for children of all ages and adults.

16. **Mag Chlor 85** is the liquid magnesium chloride that contains 85 mg per ml. Magnesium chloride is the form of magnesium that is found in the body and is best absorbed and tolerated.

17. **L–T** is a formulation that contains L-Theanine, Glutamine, and Glycine, all inhibitory amino acids. L-Theanine is a major amino acid that derives from green tea leaves. L-Theanine produces a calming effect in the brain without dulling feelings or drowsiness. Studies demonstrate that L-Theanine increases alpha waves in the brain like deep meditation. In the *Journal of Food Science & Technology* a study published confirms that theanine has a significant effect on the release of neurotransmitters such as serotonin and dopamine. L-Theanine plays a key role in the formation of GABA, an inhibitory neurotransmitter. L-Theanine also counters the effects of caffeine.

> *Remember, amino acids must be taken daily and in specific amounts for the brain to be chemically balanced.*

For product information, call 1-800-669-2256 or *visit* http://www.painstresscenter.com

A.D.D. Focus Support Program

The following is a program guide for A.D.D./A.D.H.D. focus and concentration. The program must be tailored to the individual child.

For the Little Tikes (under 50 pounds)

- **Brain Link Complex.** Follow directions according to weight, in morning and afternoon.
- *If you do not use Brain Link,* use **Little One** (non-chewable), a good children's multiple, 1 daily in AM.
- **1 DHA** (Neuromins) daily.
- **Mag Chlor 85,*** 5 to 10 drops, twice daily in juice **OR** **Calcium-Magnesium Liquid,** 1 to 2 teaspoons full per day in divided doses.
- **HTP10 Complex,**** 1 capsule 30 minutes prior to bedtime, if your child has sleep problems.
- **Liquid Serotonin** morning, afternoon, and night—1 full dropper.

Over 50 pounds, but less than 100 pounds

In the morning

- **1 SBNC** (Super Balanced Neurotransmitter Complex) cap with food **OR** 1 Brain Link serving according to weight.
- **1 AC** (Anxiety Control).
- **1 Mag Link*** **OR** if your child cannot swallow use **Mag Chlor 85,*** 10 to 15 drops, twice daily in juice **OR** **Calcium-Magnesium** liquid.

*****Special Note:*** Mag Link (ML) contains magnesium chloride, the form of magnesium found in the body. Absorption and tolerance of magnesium chloride is better than any form of magnesium. If loose stools, or diarrhea occur, reduce the amount by 1 capsule or increase interval between doses.

**DO NOT USE HTP10 or products containing 5-HTP if you are taking SSRI drugs.

• *At noon:*
- 1 AC *OR* another **Brain Link** serving.
- After school, **1 SBNC,** if needed.
- **1 DHA** or **1 ProDHA.**

Bedtime
- **HTP10 Complex,**** one (1) 30 minutes prior to bedtime.
- **Cal, Mag, Zinc** capsules as follows: 50-75 pounds, use 1 capsules; 75 to 100 pounds, use 2 capsules; 100 to 125 pounds use 3 capsules; over 150 pounds, use 4 capsules.

Over 100 pounds

First thing in the morning
- **1 T-L Vite *OR* Brain Link** according to weight.
- **2 Super Balanced Neurotransmitter Complex** (SBNC) in morning with food.
- **1 or 2 AC *OR* two (2) HTP10**** (Use HTP10** if your child exhibits anger, aggression, or depression).
- **2 Glutamine caps, *OR* 1 scoop Glutamine powder** in water or juice.
- **1 Mag Link *OR* Mag Chlor 85,** 10 to 25 drops. *

At noon
- **1 or 2 AC, *OR* 2 HTP10.****

Bedtime
- **HTP10 Complex,**** two (2) to three (3) 30 minutes prior to bedtime.
- **1 Mag Link *OR* Mag Chlor 85,** 10 to 25 drops. *
- **1 ProDHA.**

*Special Note: Mag Link (ML) contains magnesium chloride, the form of magnesium found in the body. Absorption and tolerance of magnesium chloride is better than any form of magnesium. If loose stools, or diarrhea occur, reduce the amount by 1 capsule or number of drops, or increase interval between doses.

**If your child is taking a SSRI drug, DO NOT USE 5-HTP or products containing 5-HTP.

Teen/Adult Focus

The following supports the brain for enhanced brain function, i.e. focus and concentration. The combination helps alleviate mood swings and constant carbohydrate cravings. The following combination is designed for individuals 100 pounds and over.

In the morning

- 1 **T-L Vite,** *OR* **Brain Link Complex** according to weight.
- 2 **Teen Link**** (teenagers), *OR* use **Mood Sync**** (adults).
- 2 **Glutamine caps,** *OR* 1 scoop **Glutamine powder.**
- 1 or 2 **Mag Link*** *OR* **Mag Chlor 85,*** 10 to 25 drops.
- 1 **ProDHA.**

In the afternoon

- 2 **Teen Link**** (teenagers), *OR* **Mood Sync**** (adults).
- 2 **Glutamine Caps,** *OR* 1 scoop **Super Glutamine powder.**
- 1 or 2 **Mag Link*** *OR* **Mag Chlor 85,*** 10 to 25 drops.

*Special Note: Mag Link (ML) contains magnesium chloride, the form of magnesium found in the body. Absorption and tolerance of magnesium chloride is better than any form of magnesium. If loose stools, or diarrhea occur, reduce the amount by 1 capsule or increase interval between doses.

**If your child is taking a SSRI drug, DO NOT USE 5-HTP or products containing 5-HTP.

Any of the following may be added to any program. *NOT ALL NEED TO BE ADDED.*

General health/allergies

- **Ester C,** 2,000 to 3,000 mg per day, spread throughout the day.

Concentration/memory

- **Super Glutamine,** 1 scoop daily. If over 100 pounds, use 2 scoops daily, divided **OR Glutamine caps,** 2 to 4 per day, divided.
- **HTP 10 Complex,**** use 1 or 2, twice daily for children less than 75 pounds.
- **Huperzine,** (over 12 years old) 1 capsule, twice daily.

Excessive movement

- **Taurine,** 1 to 2 (500 mg) caps, daily; teens and adults, 1 capsule (1000 mg), twice daily daily.
- **Mag Chlor 85,** dosage depends on weight.

Sleep problems/insomnia

- **Liquid Serotonin,** ½ to 1 full dropper, if less than 75 pounds. *If over 75 pounds,* use **HTP10,**** one (1) or two (2) capsules, 30 minutes prior to bedtime. *If over 150 pounds,* use 50 mg **5-HTP.*** *An alternative to pure 5-HTP*** is 1 or 2 **Teen Link**** capsules for teens OR 1 or 2 **Mood Sync**** for adults.

***Special Note:** Mag Link (ML) contains magnesium chloride, the form of magnesium found in the body. Absorption and tolerance of magnesium chloride is better than any form of magnesium. If loose stools, or diarrhea occur, reduce the amount by 1 capsule or increase interval between doses.

**If your child is taking a SSRI drug, DO NOT USE 5-HTP or products containing 5-HTP.

Sugar cravings

- **Gymnema Sylvestre,** 1 to 2 capsule daily before eating.

Picky eater

- **Brain Link** (Use as directed.) *OR*
- **BNC + GABA** powder; **glutamine powder** and **glycine** can be added, if desired.

Sinus problems

- **Xlear Nasal Spray, Sinus Allergy Spray, or Euphorbium Nasal Spray.**

Skin problems

- **Vitamin E,** 400 I.U.
- **Naturally Clear** skin formula, follow directions on package.

Gas, bloating, digestive problems

- **Kid's Digestive Enzymes,** 2 with each meal; adults use **Super Pancreatin 650,** 2 with each meal.

Pain

- Over 12 years, 1 **Pain Control** capsule.
- Apply **Pain Control Cream** topically.

For product information, call 1-800-669-2256 or visit http://www.painstresscenter.com

Special Notes

Ritalin Withdrawal

If your child is taking Ritalin, Adderall, or Cylert and you wish to start a withdrawal program, Ron Lopez, M.D., Orthomolecular Psychiatrist suggests the following schedule.

1) Begin a daily amino acids and nutrient program before you reduce his Ritalin or any prescription drug.
2) First stop the drug on the weekends.
3) Reduce the dosage by one-half for two weeks.
4) Reduce the dosage again by one-half for one week.
5) Then discontinue completely.
6) Use orthomolecular therapy to support the brain throughout.
7) Establish your child's amino acid imbalances and continue to supply nutritional support.

Pycnogenol

Over the past several months my staff has received numerous phone calls from concerned parents regarding the use of Pycnogenol for A.D.D. and A.D.H.D. children.

Pycnogenol is an antioxidant that has numerous benefits. Pycnogenol can improve circulation and, hence, oxygenation of brain tissue, but it does not create needed neurotransmitters in the brain which A.D.D. and A.D.H.D. children desperately need. Yes, children taking Pycnogenol may show some improvement, but that is a given when you take an antioxidant such as Pycnogenol. For a child to concentrate, focus, and stay on task, he or she must follow a complete orthomolecular program that contains inhibitory amino acids that create neurotransmitters.

Enzymes

Kids need enzymes, too. Every organ in the body needs enzymes for normal functioning. Every organ system of the body requires enzymes in order to perform our daily activities and keep us alive. Enzymes support the body's defenses and immune system.

Children can suffer from enzyme deficiency just like adults, since both eat diets deficient in enzymes. Enzymes are safe for children and have no side effects. If you start plant enzyme supplementation at an early age, you help preserve the enzyme potential of the child. The enzyme-making potential gives the child's organs the ability to make either digestive or metabolic enzymes. If your child uses too much of his enzymes to manufacture digestive enzymes, then the metabolic enzymes production is limited—and your child becomes more susceptible to digestive disorders, a weakened immune system, and disease. Children with allergies often require enzymes to support their digestive tract, organs and defenses.

Benefits of Digestive Enzymes
- Improved digestion, nutrient assimilation, and enhanced nutrient absorption.
- Improved digestion of proteins (amino acids).
- Disease prevention.
- Does not interfere with medication.
- Corrects digestion to stop gas, bloating, bowel problems, heartburn, food allergies, and fatigue after eating.

Amino Acids for Brain and Body Function

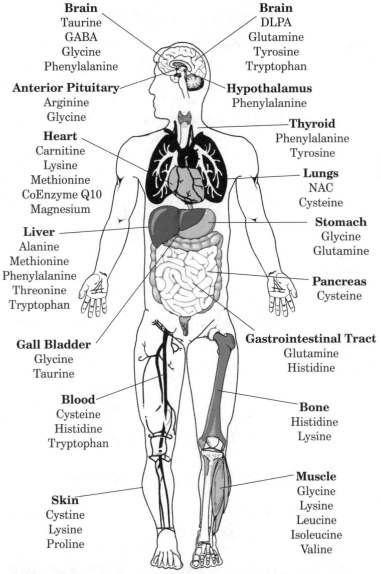

Brain
Taurine
GABA
Glycine
Phenylalanine

Brain
DLPA
Glutamine
Tyrosine
Tryptophan

Anterior Pituitary
Arginine
Glycine

Hypothalamus
Phenylalanine

Thyroid
Phenylalanine
Tyrosine

Heart
Carnitine
Lysine
Methionine
CoEnzyme Q10
Magnesium

Lungs
NAC
Cysteine

Liver
Alanine
Methionine
Phenylalanine
Threonine
Tryptophan

Stomach
Glycine
Glutamine

Pancreas
Cysteine

Gall Bladder
Glycine
Taurine

Gastrointestinal Tract
Glutamine
Histidine

Blood
Cysteine
Histidine
Tryptophan

Bone
Histidine
Lysine

Muscle
Glycine
Lysine
Leucine
Isoleucine
Valine

Skin
Cystine
Lysine
Proline

Always add magnesium and B6 or P5'P to all amino acids.

*For more information about amino acids,
read my book Heal with Amino Acids*

Common Symptoms of Food Allergies

Physical Symptoms

Skin	Hives, rash, eczema, dermatitis, pallor.
Head	Insomnia, fainting spells, headaches, dizziness, feeling of fullness in the head, excessive drowsiness or sleepiness soon after eating.
Eyes, Ears, Nose, and Throat	Stuffy nose, runny nose, excessive mucous formation, post nasal drip, watery eyes, earache, fullness of ears, fluid in the middle ear, hearing loss, recurrent ear infections, itching ear, ear drainage, sore throats, chronic cough, gagging, canker sores, itching of the roof of the mouth, recurrent sinusitis.
Heart and Lungs	Increased heart rate, asthma, palpitations, congestion in the chest, arrhythmias, tachycardia.
Gastrointestinal	Nausea, vomiting, diarrhea, constipation, bloating after meals, belching, colitis, flatulence (passing gas), feeling of fullness in the stomach long after finishing a meal, abdominal pains or cramps.
Other Symptoms	Chronic fatigue, weakness, muscle aches and pains, joint aches and pains, arthritis, swelling of the hands, feet or ankles, urinary tract symptoms such as frequency of urination or urgency, vaginal itching, vaginal discharge, hunger, *binge or spree* eating.

Psychological Symptoms

Anxiety, panic attacks, depression, crying jags, aggressive behavior, irritability, mental dullness, mental lethargy, confusion, excessive daydreaming, hyperactivity, restlessness, learning disabilities, poor work habits, slurred speech, stuttering, inability to concentrate, indifference.

Various Foods Known To Cause Allergies

Almond
Apple
Apricot
Arrowroot
Artichoke
Asparagus
Banana
Beans
Beef
Beet
Blueberry
Brazil nut
Broccoli
Brussels sprouts
Buckwheat
Cabbage
Carrot
Cashew
Cauliflower
Celery
Cherry
Chicken ·
Chocolate
Citrus fruits
Clam
Cloves
Cocoa
Coconut
Coffee
Corn
Cranberry

Cucumber
Currant
Eggs
Eggplant
Figs
Fish, all types
Garlic
Ginger
Gooseberry
Grapes
Leeks
Lemons
Lentils
Lettuce
Mango
Melons
Milk ·
Mushrooms
Mustard
Nuts
Oats
Okra
Olives
Onions
Oranges
Oysters
Peaches
Peas
Peanuts
Pecans

Peppers (red or green)
Persimmons
Pineapple
Plums
Pork
Potato, white ·
Prunes
Pumpkin
Rhubarb
Rice
Sassafras
Scallops
Seafood
Shrimp
Soy products
Spices
Spinach
Squash
Strawberries
Sweet potato
Sugar
Tapioca
Tomatoes
Turkey
Turnips
Vanilla
Walnuts
Wheat
Wintergreen
Yeast

Signs And Symptoms of Cow's Milk Allergy

Gastrointestinal

Abdominal pain
Abdominal distention
Colic in infants
Colitis (inflammation of colon)
Constipation
Stomachache
Diarrhea
Gas
Heartburn
Indigestion
Intestinal obstruction (infants)
Malabsorption
Mouth ulcers
Peptic ulcers
Poor appetite
Rectal bleeding
Vomiting

Respiratory

Asthma
Bronchitis
Cough
Croup
Earache
Frequent colds
Hair loss
Nasal congestion
Nose bleeds
Recurrent pneumonia
Postnasal drip
Runny nose
Sinusitis
Sore throat
Stuffy nose
Wheezing

Miscellaneous

Red eyes due to allergy
Anaphylaxis
Anemia
Arthritis-like symptoms
Bad breath
Bed-wetting
Behavior disorders
Cardiac irregularities
Right heart failure
Cystitis
Excessive sweating
Failure to thrive
Fatigue
"Growing pains"
Headache
Heart disease
Hyperactivity
Irritability
Lassitude
Vaginal discharge
Migraine
Musculoskeletal pain
Nephritic syndrome
Paleness
Pallor
Polyarthritis
Tension
Thrombocytopenia

Skin/Dermatological

Acne
Swollen lips
Dark circles around eyes
Eczema
Hives

Source: *Food Allergies Made Simple* by Phylis Austin et. al

Warning Signs of Inadequate Nutrition

Organ Systems	Physical Signs	Nutrient Deficiency
Neck	Goiter	Iodine
Teeth	Dental cavities	Fluoride
	Mottled enamel	Excess Fluoride
	Cavities	Vitamin C Phosphorus
	Malposition	Protein-calorie
Tongue	Red, painful sore	B6 (Pyridoxine) Folic Acid
	Swollen	Iron
	Purple	Riboflavin
	Scarlet, raw	Niacin
Mouth	Sore, cracked and chapped lips	Riboflavin
Face	Brown, patchy pigmentation of cheeks. Parotid enlargement, *moon* face	Protein-calorie
Lips	Inflammation of the mucus membranes of the lips	Riboflavin
Nose	Whiteheads and blackheads along border of nose and cheeks.	B6 (Pyridoxine)
Gums	Hypertrophy or overgrowth of gums	Vitamin C
	Inflammation of gums	Vitamin A Niacin Riboflavin
Eyes	Extreme sensitivity to light, poor twilight vision, loss of shine, bright and moist appearance, loss of light reflex, decreased tears, softening of the cornea.	Vitamin A
	Paleness inside of eyelid.	Iron or folate
	Moist and red tissues at external angles of both eyes.	Riboflavin

Nails	Ridging, brittle, easily broken, flattened, spoon-shaped, thin, lusterless.	Iron
√ **Hair**	Becomes dull, fine, brittle, straight. Becomes red in Blacks, then lighter in color, may be bleached in Whites, easily and pain-lessly pluckable; outer one-third of eyebrow may be sparse in hypothyroidsim (cretinism, iodine deficiency, or other).	Protein-calorie
Skin	Dryness of skin, follicular hyperkeratosis (*gooseflesh, sandpaper skin,* acne lesions).	Vitamins A, E
	Red spots that produce *pink halo* effects around coiled follicles, purple bruises in skin due to capillary fragility, bleeds into joints, cortical hemorrhages of bone visible on x-ray.	Vitamin C
	Hemorrhages in skin, gastrointestinal	Vitamin K
	Pallor, jaundice.	Vitamin B12
	Pallor	Iron
	Redness of skin occurring in patches of vari-able sizes and shape early, then vasculariza-tion, crusting, shedding, increased pigmen-tation; thickened, inelastic fissures in skin, especially in skin exposed to skin, becoming scaly; dry pigmentation, of the cheek and above the eye.	Niacin
Skeletal	Osteoporosis (in association with low protein and fluoride deficiency).	Calcium
	Growth part of bone is enlarged, *beating* ribs, delayed fusion of cranial fontanels, bowed legs, deformities of thorax (such as pigeon breast), osteomalacia in adults.	Vitamin D
	Hematoma in bone, enlargement of the growth part of bones, painless.	Vitamin C
Muscular	Loss of tone.	Vitamin D
	Muscle wasting, weakness, fatigue, inactivity, loss of subcutaneous fat.	Protein-calorie
	Accumulation of blood within the muscles.	Vitamin C
	Calf muscle tenderness, weakness.	Thiamine
Central Nervous System (CNS)	Apathy, irritability, psychomotor changes	Protein
	Psychotic behavior (dementia).	Niacin

Central Nervous System CNS) **(Continued)**	Peripheral neuropathy, symmetrical sensory and motor deficits, especially in lower extremities; drug resistant convulsions (infants), dementia, forgetful.	B6 (Pyridoxine)
	Lack of reflexes, loss of position and vibratory senses, tingling of skin.	Vitamin B12
	Tremors, convulsions, behavioral disturbances.	Magnesium (magnesium chloride)
Liver	Fatty infiltration of liver.	Protein-calorie
Gastrointestinal (GI)	Anorexia, flatulence, diarrhea.	Vitamin B12
	Anorexia.	Zinc
	Diarrhea	Niacin, Protein-calorie
Cardiovascular	Rapid heartbeat, congestive heart failure, heart enlargement, electro-cardiographic changes (EKG).	Thiamine CoEnzyme Q10 Magnesium (magnesium chloride)

Process for Establishing Vitamin Requirements for the Human Body
(Children and Adults)

- Amount required to prevent symptoms of a deficiency.
- Amount required to saturate body tissues.
- Amount required to produce maximum blood levels.
- Amount required to produce maximum activity of an enzyme.
- Actual amount of vitamins used by an individual on a daily basis.
- Amount required to replace needed nutrients in those with food allergies.

Criteria established by the *National Institute of Health*.

Bibliography

Adams, Ruth and Frank Murray. *Megavitamin Therapy.* New York: Larchmont Books, 1980.

Agren, H. et al. "Low brain uptake of L-5-hydroxytryptophan in major depression: A positron emission tomography study on patients and healthy volunteers. *Acta Psychiatry Scan.* Vol. 83, 1991, pp. 449–455.

American Journal of Disease of Children, December 16–21, 1985.

Armstrong, Thomas. *The Myth of the A.D.D. Child,* New York: Penquin Books, 1995.

Appleton, Nancy. Lick the Sugar Habit. Garden City Park, NY: Avery Publishing Group, 1996.

Angst J. et al. "The treatment of depression with l-5-hydroxytryptophan versus imipramine: Results of two open and one double-blind study. *Arch Psychiatry Nervenkr.* Vol. 224, 1977, pp. 175–186.

Austin, Phylis, Thrash, Agatha, and Thrash, Calvin. *Food Allergies Made Simple.* Seale, AL: New Lifestyle Books, 1985.

Balch, James F. and Phyllis A. Balch. *Prescription for Nutritional Healing: A-to-Z Guide to Supplements.* Garden City Park, NY, 1998.

Bland, Jeffrey. *Medical Applications of Clinical Nutrition.* New Canaan, Conn: Keats Publishing, Inc., 1983.

Breggin, Peter R. *Talking Back to Prozac.* New York: St. Martin's Press, 1994.

Breggin, Peter R. *Toxic Psychiatry,* New York: St. Martin's Press, 1991.

Breggin, Peter R. and Ginger R. Breggin. *The War Against Children,* New York, St. Martin's Press, 1994.

Carey, William B. "A Suggested Solution to the Confusion in Attention Deficit Diagnoses." *Clinical Pediatrics.* Vol. 27, No. 7, July, 1988, pp. 348–349.

Children's Health. (Entire Issue) *Complementary Medicine.* Vol. 3, No. 2, Winter, 1988.

Cohen, Sidney. *The Chemical Brain, The Neurochemistry of Addictive Disorders.* Irvine, CA: Care Institute, 1988.

Cooper, Jack R., Floyd E. Bloom, and Robert H. *The Biochemical Basis of Neuropharmacology.* New York: Oxford University Press, 1986.

Cooper, Remi. *The Essential Omega 3 Fatty Acid DHA.* Pleasant Grove,

UT: Woodland Publishing, 1998.

Cott, Allan. *The Orthomolecular Approach to Learning Disabilities.* Novato, CA: Academic Therapy Publications, 1977.

Cott, Allan, Jerome Agel, and Eugene Boe. *Dr. Cott's Help Your Learning Disabled Child.* New York: Times Books, Random House, 1985.

Crook, William G. and Laura Stevens. *Solving the Puzzle of Your Hard-To-Raise Child.* New York: Vintage Books, 1988.

Essman, W.B., ed. *Nutrients and Brain Function.* New York: Karger Publishers, 1987.

"Experts Disagree on Use of Ritalin in A.D.D. Treatment." *C.N.N. Today,* November 2, 1995.

Feingold, Ben F. *Why Your Child is Hyperactive.* New York: Random House, 1974.

"Fish Oils, Bones, and Joints." Nutrition Alert. Nov./Dec. 2001, p. 8.

Gitlin, Michael J. *The Psychotherapist's Guide to Psychopharmacology.* New York: The Free Press, 1990.

Glenmullen, Joseph. *Prozac Backlash.* New York: Simon & Schuster, 2000.

Graedon and Teresa Graedon. *The People's Guide to Deadly Drug Interactions.* New York: St. Martin's Press, 1995.

Green, Wayne H. *Child and Adolescent Clinical Psychopharmacology.* Baltimore: Williams and Wilkins, 1991.

Grollman, Earl A. *Talking About Death.* Boston: Beacon Press, 1976.

Hamburg, Beatrix A. "Early Adolescence." *Postgraduate Medicine.* Vol. 78, No. 1, July, 1985, pp. 158–172.

Hart, Carol. *Secrets of Serotonin.* New York: St. Martin Press, 1996.

Hoffer, Abram and Morton Walker. *Orthomolecular Nutrition New Lifestyle for Super Good Health.* New Canaan, CN: Keats Publishing, Inc., 1978.

Irwin, M., K. Belendiuk, K. McCloskey, et al. "Tryptophan Metabolism in Children with Attentional Deficit Disorder." *American Journal of Psychiatry.* Vol. 138, No. 8, pp. 1082–1085.

Kotulak, Ronald. *Inside the Brain.* Kansas City: Andrews and McMeel, 1996.

Ledoux, Joseph. *Synaptic Self: How Our Brains Become Who We Are.* New York: Penquin Putnam, 2002.

Leonard, B.E. *Fundamentals of Psychopharmacology.* New York: John Wiley & Sons, 1992.

Lininger, Skye, ed. *The Natural Pharmacy.* Rocklin, CA: Prima

Publishing, 1998.

Lopez, D.A., R.M. Williams, and K. Miehlke. *Enzymes: The Fountain of Life.* The Neville Press, Inc., 1994, p. 1.

Martin, Paul. "Helping for the Learning Disabled." *Health Express.* June, 1983, pp. 78–79.

Moore, Thomas J. *Prescription for Disaster: The Hidden Dangers in Your Medicine Cabinet.* New York: Simon & Schuster, 1998.

Mowrey, Daniel. *Herbal Tonic Therapies.* New Canaan, CT: Keats Publishing, 1993.

New York Times, May 5, 1987, p. 3.

Murray, Michael. *Boost Your Serotonin Levels, 5-HTP.* New York: Bantam Books, 1998.

Nardini, M., et al. "Treatment of depression with l-5-hydroxytryptophan combined with clomipramine: A double blind study. *Journal Clinical Pharmacology Research.* Vol. 2, 1983, pp. 239–250.

Norden, Michael. *Beyond Prozac.* New York, NY: Harper Collins, 1995.

Passwater, Richard A. and James South. *5-HTP: The Natural Serotonin Solution.* New Canaan, CT: Keats Publishing, 1988.

Pfeiffer, Carl. *Nutrition and Mental Illness, An Orthomolecular Approach to Balancing Body Chemistry.* Rochester, VT: Healing Arts Press, 1987.

Phelps, Janice Keller and Nourse, Alan E. *The Hidden Addiction and How to Get Free.* Boston: Little, Brown and Company, 1986.

Podell, Richard N. "Food, Mind, and Mood, Hyperactivity Revisited." *Postgraduate Medicine.* Vol. 78, No. 2, August, 1985, pp. 119–125.

Pollock, Ellen J. "Managed Care's Focus on Psychiatric Drugs Alarms Many Doctors," *Wall Street Journal,* December 1, 1995.

Rapp. Doris J. *Allergies and the Hyperactive Child.* New York: Simon and Schuster, Inc., 1979.

Rapp, Doris J. *Is This Your Child?* New York: William Morrow and Company, Inc., 1991.

Rapp., Doris J. *Is This Your Child's World?* New York: Bantam, 1997.

The Reporter Weekly. September 2, 1987, p. 10.

Rogers, L.L. and R. B. Pelton. "Effect of Glutamine on I.Q. Scores of Mentally Deficient Children." *Texas Reports on Biology and Medicine.* Vol. 15, No. 1, 1957.

Safer, D. J. and J.M. Krager. "A Survey of Medication Treatment for Hyperactive/Inattentive Students." *Journal of the American*

Medical Association. October 21, 1988, Vol. 260, No. 15, pp. 2256–2258.

Sahley, Billie and Katherine M. Birkner. *Breaking Your Prescribed Addiction.* San Antonio, TX: Pain & Stress Publications, 1998.

Sahley, Billie. *GABA, The Anxiety Amino Acid.* San Antonio, TX: Pain & Stress Publications, 2001.

Sahley, Billie and Katherine M. Birkner. *Heal with Amino Acids,* San Antonio: Pain & Stress Publications, 2001.

Sahley, Billie. *Is Ritalin Necessary? The Ritalin Report.* San Antonio, TX: Pain & Stress Publications, 2001.

Sahley, Billie. *Post Trauma and Chronic Emotional Fatigue.* San Antonio, TX: Pain & Stress Publications, 2002.

Sahley, Billie. *The Anxiety Epidemic.* San Antonio, TX: Pain & Stress Publications, 2002.

Shaywitz, S.E. and Shaywitz, B.A. "Increased Medication Use in Attention-Deficit Hyperactivity Disorder: Regressive or Appropriate?" *Journal of the American Medical Association.* October 21, 1988, Vol. 260, No. 15, pp. 2270–2272.

Shute, Wilfrid. *Health Preserver, Defining the Versatility of Vitamin E.* Emmanus, PA: Rodale Press, 1977.

Smith, Lendon. *Feed Your Kids Right.* New York: Dell Publishing, 1988.

Smith, Lendon. *Improving Your Child's Behavior Chemistry.* New York: Simon & Schuster, 1977.

Schatzberg, Alan F. and Charles B. Nemeroff, ed. *Textbook of Psychopharmacology.* Washington, D.C.: American Psychiatric Press, Inc., 1995.

Stewart, Mark. *Raising A Hyperactive Child.* New York: Harper Row, 1973.

Thomas, Karen. "Ritalin's Makers' Ties to Advocate Probed," *USA Today,* November 16, 1995.

USA Today. Newslines, October 28, 1988, Section A, p.1.

Williams, R.J. *Alcoholism: The Nutritional Approach.* Austin, TX: University of Texas Press, 1958.

Williams, Roger. *Biochemical Individuality.* Austin, TX: University of Texas Press, 1979.

Wilson, Eva D., Katherine H. Fisher, and Pilar A. Garcia. *Principles of Nutrition.* New York: John Wiley & Sons, 1979.

World News Tonight with Peter Jennings. *ABC News,* February 15, 1995.

Wunderlich, Ray C, Jr. and Dwight K. Kalita. *Nourishing Your Child: A Bioecologic Approach.* New Canaan, CN: Keats Publishing, Inc., 1984.

Index

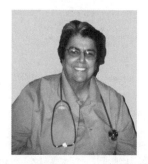

About the Author

Billie J. Sahley, Ph.D., is Executive Director of the Pain & Stress Center in San Antonio. She is a Board Certified Medical Psychotherapist & Psychodiagnostician, Behavior Therapist, and an Orthomolecular Therapist. She is a Diplomate in the American Academy of Pain Management. Dr. Sahley is a graduate of the University of Texas, Clayton University School of Behavioral Medicine, and U.C.L.A. School of Integral Medicine. Additionally, she has studied advanced nutritional biochemistry through Jeffrey Bland, Ph.D., Director of HealthComm. She is a member of the Huxley Foundation/Academy of Orthomolecular Medicine, American Academy of Environmental Medicine, Academy of Psychosomatic Medicine, North American Nutrition and Preventive Medicine Association, and American Counseling Association. In addition, she holds memberships in the Sports Medicine Foundation, American Association of Hypnotherapists, and American Mental Health Counselors Association. She also sits on the Scientific and Medical Advisory Board for Inter-Cal Corporation.

Dr. Sahley wrote: *The Anxiety Epidemic; GABA, The Anxiety Amino Acid; Post Trauma and Chronic Emotional Fatigue; Malic Acid and Magnesium For Fibromyalgia and Chronic Pain Syndrome; The Melatonin Report; Is Ritalin Necessary? The Ritalin Report;* and has recorded numerous audiocassette tapes. She coauthored *Breaking Your Prescribed Addiction, and Heal With Amino Acids.*

In addition, Dr. Sahley holds three U.S. patents for: SAF, Calms Kids (SAF For Kids), and Anxiety Control 24. Dr. Sahley devotes the majority of her time to research, writing, and development of natural products to address brain deficiencies.